Anti-Alzheimer's Cooking

An Alzheimer's Cookbook for All Novices

BY - Ana Rose

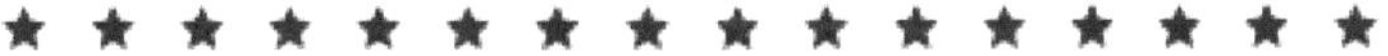

★ ★ ★ ★ ★ ★ ★ ★ ★ ★ ★ ★ ★ ★ ★ ★ ★ ★

Copyrighting Notice

As a gentlewoman, kindly refrain from selling, publishing, printing, copying, disseminating or distributing the contents of this book. Such actions can only be allowed by the author. If perchance you have obtained an unauthorized copy, it is requested that you delete it without delay and purchase the legal version.

It is important to note that the author cannot be held liable for any actions taken by the reader based on the information provided in this book. This publication serves as an informational tool and the author has taken every measure to ensure the accuracy of the information. Therefore, any steps taken based on the contents must be approached with prudence.

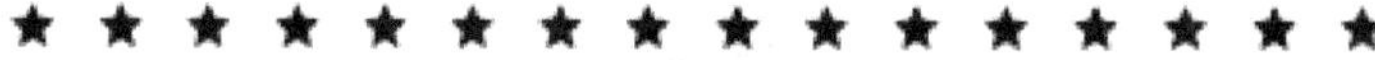

Table of Contents

Introduction

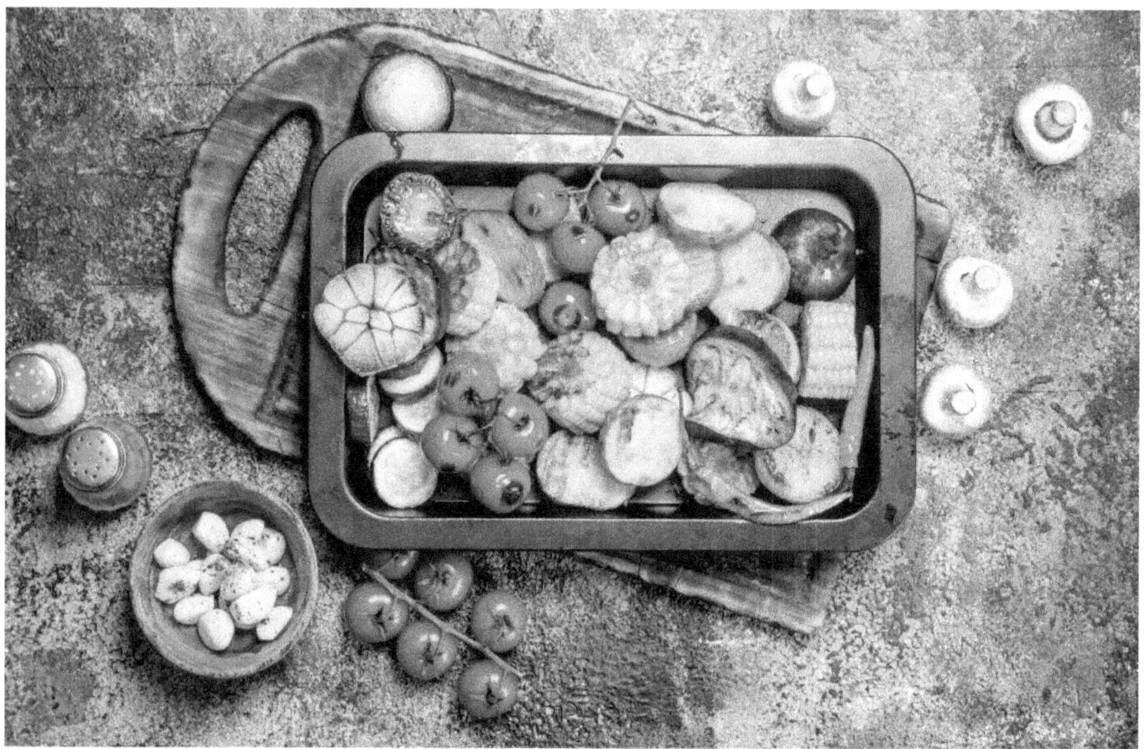

Sitting majestically atop our spinal column resides our incredible command central, an intricate masterpiece interlinking each bodily necessity under governing rule. The encircling cortex houses critical links to memory, while dynamic messengers travel along neural superhighways, fueling mobility, perception, and sensory delight. It mind-boggles scholars still attempting a full description of this regulator supreme, where even slight disruptions can greatly hinder the entire system's harmony! How incredibly miraculous it is that we get to experience such divine genius controlling our mere mortal frames!

Always operative yet mysteriously obscured behind skull walls, the human brain remains perpetually active, necessitating constant sustenance. Comparatively likening its operation to that of an airplane highlights the importance of varied substances to optimize performance and avoid detrimental consequences stemming from subpar energy sources. Even though the brain functions during periods of slumber and may ingest less than optimal sustenance, it deserves premium quality nourishing essentials that support sustained peak efficiency. Just as an airplane requires meticulously formulated fuels and lubricants to maintain aerial competency and prolong longevity, so too does the marvelous thinking machine thrive on targeted supportive sustenance.

Alzheimer's debilitates crucial neurological processes in the cerebrum. Preclinical phases emerging roughly ten years prior to visible indicators should raise urgent concern. Accelerated accumulation of protein aggregates, including amyloid plaque buildup and tau entanglements, accompany declining cognitive abilities. Worsening conditions cause irreversible cell death, triggering profound shrinkage. Tragic cascading consequences wreak havoc on functional gray matter, mandating dedicated countermeasures prior to severe stages.

Just like an aircraft running on car fuel, if your brain doesn't have the necessary nutrients for its complex functions, it will stumble.

sssssssssssssssssss

1. Honey Salmon Steaks with a Sesame Rocket Salad

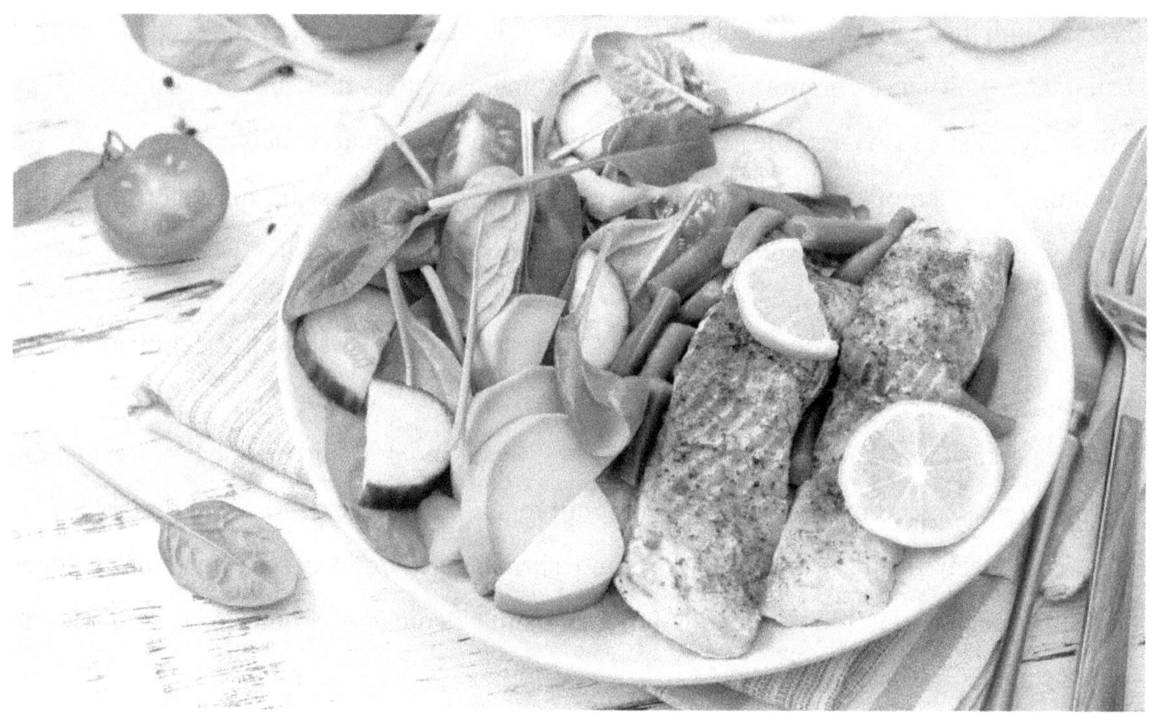

This is a light recipe but you have to be very quick in it. By mixing honey and olive oil together, the salmon will take the flavor of the honey - you will be very surprised with the result. You can do the same with herbs such as thyme and coriander as well.

Serve: 4

Prep Time: 20 minutes

List of Ingredients:

- 2 tablespoons of sesame seeds
- 1 bag of rocket salad
- 1 lemon, cut into quarters for garnish
- 4 salmon steak
- 2 tablespoons of lemon juice
- 3 tablespoons of olive oil
- 3 tablespoons of honey

sssssssssssssssssss

Methods:

Step 1: Prepare the Salmon

Begin by warming up the olive oil in a frying pan over medium heat. The gentle heat will ensure the salmon cooks evenly without burning.

Once the oil is warmed, add the honey to the pan. Mix the honey well with the oil to create a sweet and savory glaze for the salmon.

Step 2: Cook the Salmon Steaks

When the oil is sufficiently hot, carefully place the salmon steaks into the pan, skin side down. This will help achieve a crispy skin.

Allow the salmon to cook for about 3 to 4 minutes on each side, adjusting the time based on the thickness of your salmon. The salmon should turn a beautiful golden color and flake easily when cooked.

Step 3: Prepare the Sesame Rocket Salad

While the salmon is cooking, prepare the rocket salad. Take a large serving bowl and place the fresh rocket leaves in it. Rocket, also known as arugula, has a peppery and slightly bitter flavor that pairs well with the salmon's sweetness.

Step 4: Toast Sesame Seeds and Deglaze

Once the salmon steaks are done cooking, remove them from the heat and keep them warm.

In the same frying pan, add the sesame seeds and cook them for 1 to 2 minutes until they become fragrant and slightly golden. This toasting process enhances the nutty flavor of the seeds.

Quickly deglaze the pan by pouring in the lemon juice. The lemon juice will lift up the flavorful bits from the bottom of the pan and create a tangy sauce.

Step 5: Assemble the Salad

Pour the sesame seed and lemon juice dressing onto the rocket salad. The combination of the toasted sesame and tangy lemon will create a well-balanced dressing.

Mix the salad thoroughly to coat the rocket leaves evenly with the dressing. Take a moment to season the salad with a pinch of salt and freshly ground black pepper, enhancing the flavors.

Step 6: Serve the Dish

You're now ready to serve this delightful dish. Place the honey-glazed salmon steaks either on top of the rocket salad or on the side, depending on your preference.

The contrast between the warm, succulent salmon and the crisp, peppery rocket salad creates a harmonious blend of textures and flavors.

Fun Facts:

Salmon is an excellent source of omega-3 fatty acids, which are known to be beneficial for heart health and brain function.

Sesame seeds not only add a delightful crunch to the salad but also provide essential minerals like calcium and iron.

The peppery flavor of rocket leaves, also known as arugula, is not only delicious but also believed to have natural detoxifying properties that can aid digestion.

Suggestions:

For a burst of freshness, consider adding some diced avocado or orange segments to the rocket salad.

To elevate the presentation, garnish the dish with a sprinkle of freshly chopped herbs like parsley or chives.

For an extra crunch, add some crushed nuts, such as toasted almonds or pine nuts, to the rocket salad just before serving.

To add an extra layer of flavor, drizzle a bit of balsamic glaze over the salmon before serving.

2. Minted Pesto Lamb Salad

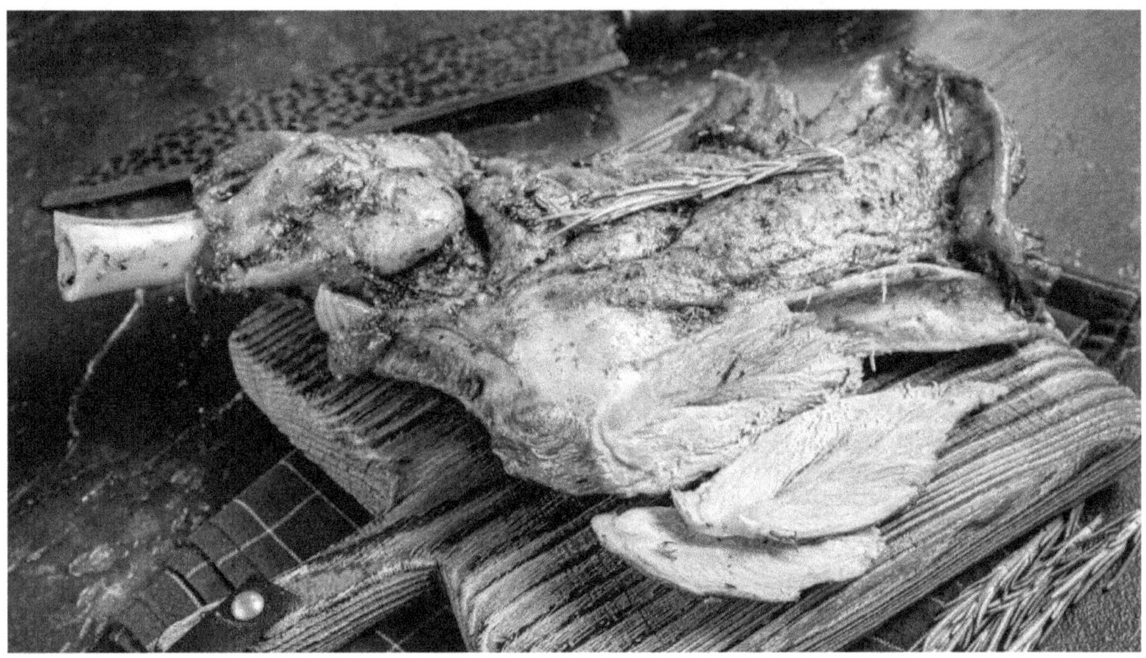

Make sure you make enough minted pesto dressing since people always ask for more. The lamb must be pink and cold but you can always have it warm too. The same for the peppers. Cook longer if you prefer tender and not crunchy.

Serve: 4

Prep Time: 20 minutes

List of Ingredients:

- 2 garlic cloves, crushed
- 1 salad of your choice
- 2 tablespoons of pine nuts
- 2 oz. of fresh basil
- ½ cup of olive oil
- Salt and pepper
- 5 lb. Of lamb, cooked and sliced
- 1 onion, sliced
- 1 red pepper, cut into strips
- 1 yellow pepper, cut into strips
- 1 oz. of fresh mints

SSSSSSSSSSSSSSSSSSSS

Methods:

Step 1: Prepare the Salad Base

Begin by preparing your choice of salad in a large bowl. Opt for fresh greens like spinach, arugula, or mixed lettuces. These greens provide a crisp and nutritious base for your lamb salad.

Step 2: Add Peppers and Onion

Dice red and yellow peppers to add vibrant colors and a sweet crunch to your salad.

Incorporate finely chopped onion for a mild and slightly tangy flavor. Mixing the onion well with the peppers and salad greens adds complexity to each bite.

Step 3: Create the Minted Pesto

In a blender, combine the pine nuts, basil leaves, and mint leaves. The pine nuts provide a creamy texture, while the basil and mint contribute aromatic and fresh herbal notes.

Season the mixture with a pinch of salt and freshly ground black pepper to enhance the flavors.

Start blending the ingredients, gradually adding olive oil in small increments. This step ensures the pesto achieves a smooth and consistent texture.

Step 4: Assemble the Salad

Divide the prepared salad mixture into four portions and arrange them on individual plates. The bed of fresh greens creates a visually appealing foundation for the dish.

Step 5: Add Slices of Lamb

Place slices of cooked lamb on top of each portion of the salad. The tender and flavorful lamb adds protein and richness to the dish, complementing the freshness of the greens.

Step 6: Drizzle with Minted Pesto

Drizzle a generous amount of the prepared minted pesto over each plate. The combination of pine nuts, basil, and mint in the pesto will infuse the dish with a burst of fragrant flavors.

Step 7: Serve and Enjoy

Your Minted Pesto Lamb Salad is now ready to be savored. The harmonious blend of flavors and textures creates a delightful and satisfying dish.

Serve this salad as a main course for a light and refreshing lunch or dinner option.

Fun Facts:

Mint is known for its refreshing and aromatic qualities, which can add a unique twist to traditional pesto flavors.

Did you know that lamb is a great source of protein and is often enjoyed in various cuisines around the world?

Mint has been used for centuries not only in culinary applications but also for its potential health benefits, including aiding digestion and providing relief from indigestion.

Suggestions:

Enhance the flavors of the salad by adding a handful of crumbled feta cheese for a creamy and tangy element.

For a burst of sweetness and texture, include pomegranate arils or dried cranberries in the salad.

To enhance the visual appeal, garnish the plates with additional fresh basil leaves or mint sprigs for a pop of color and a hint of fragrance.

For added texture, sprinkle some toasted sesame seeds or chopped nuts, such as pistachios or almonds, over the salad just before serving.

If you have any leftover minted pesto, store it in an airtight container in the refrigerator. It can be used as a versatile condiment for other dishes.

After enjoying your delicious salad, clean the blender, bowls, and utensils promptly to maintain a tidy cooking space.

3. Grilled Chicken with Endives, Cashew Salad

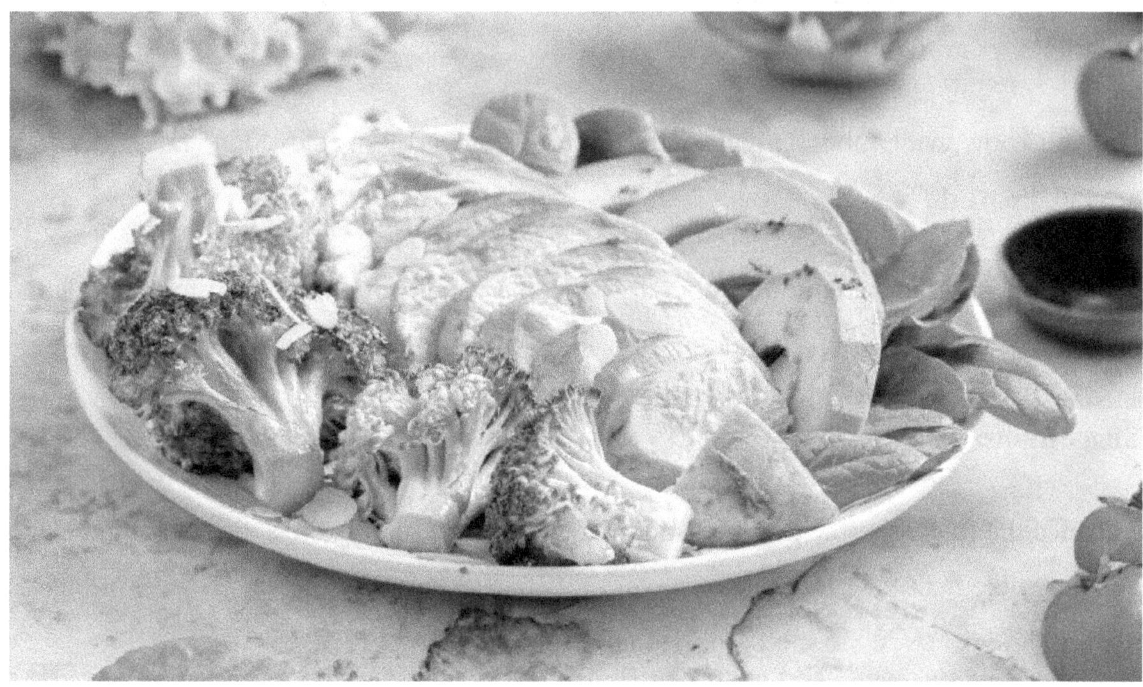

The endive is a particularly low-calorie leafy vegetable. It is a good source of minerals and it is particularly useful for pregnant women or women who wish to conceive. You can either eat it raw or cooked, as a salad or in "gratin" bake.

Serve: 4

Prep Time: 35 minutes

List of Ingredients:

- 2 tablespoons of olive oil
- 1 red onion, sliced
- 1 cup of unsalted cashew
- ¼ cup of lemon juice
- ¼ cup of coriander, chopped
- Salt and pepper
- 2 endives, shredded
- ½ a cos lettuce, shredded
- 4 chicken breasts
- 1 cup of dry raisins
- 1 cup of yogurt
- 2 garlic cloves, finely chopped

ssssssssssssssssss

Methods:

Step 1: Prepare and Flatten the Chicken

Begin by flattening the chicken breasts using a kitchen hammer or a rolling pin. Flattening the chicken ensures even cooking and allows for a quicker grilling time.

Gently pound the chicken to an even thickness, about 1/2 to 3/4 inch, to promote uniform cooking.

Step 2: Brush with Olive Oil

Brush the flattened chicken breasts with olive oil. This not only adds flavor but also prevents the chicken from sticking to the grill.

Step 3: Grill the Chicken

Place the oiled chicken breasts under the grill (or on a grill pan) and cook until they are thoroughly done. Cooking time will vary depending on the thickness of the chicken, but a good indicator is when the internal temperature reaches 165°F (75°C).

Ensure the chicken is well-cooked while retaining its juiciness. Grilling imparts a smoky flavor that compliments the salad's fresh ingredients.

Step 4: Prepare the Yogurt Dressing

In a bowl, combine the yogurt, minced garlic, fresh lemon juice, and chopped coriander (also known as cilantro). These ingredients come together to create a flavorful and tangy dressing for the salad.

Mix the dressing well to ensure all the flavors are evenly distributed, and then set it aside.

Step 5: Combine Endives and Lettuce

In a large serving bowl, combine the endives and cos (romaine) lettuce. The mixture of these two greens adds both bitterness and crunch to the salad, creating a dynamic texture.

Step 6: Add Toppings

Incorporate finely sliced red onion, cashew nuts, and raisins into the bowl. These toppings provide a variety of flavors and textures, making each bite enjoyable.

Toss the ingredients gently to combine them, ensuring an even distribution of flavors.

Step 7: Dress the Salad

Drizzle the prepared yogurt dressing over the salad mixture. The creamy yogurt balances the bitterness of the endives and adds a refreshing element to the dish.

Gently toss the salad to ensure all the ingredients are coated with the dressing.

Step 8: Assemble and Serve

To serve, slice the grilled chicken into strips and arrange them on top of the dressed salad. The warm chicken provides a hearty protein component to the dish.

Your Grilled Chicken with Endives and Cashew Salad is now ready to be enjoyed. The combination of flavors, textures, and colors creates a satisfying and nutritious meal.

Fun Facts:

Endives, also known as chicory, are a great source of fiber and provide a slightly bitter flavor that adds complexity to salads.

Cashews not only add a delicious nutty crunch to the salad but also provide healthy fats and essential nutrients.

Coriander, also known as cilantro, is an herb that offers a unique citrusy and slightly peppery flavor profile, making it a versatile addition to various dishes.

Suggestions:

Enhance the flavors of the salad by adding crumbled feta or goat cheese for a creamy and tangy contrast.

For a burst of sweetness, consider adding diced fresh mango or pomegranate arils to the salad.

To add a hint of heat, consider adding a pinch of red chili flakes to the yogurt dressing.

For added protein, include some sliced avocado or boiled eggs on top of the salad.

If you have any leftover salad or yogurt dressing, store them separately in airtight containers in the refrigerator.

After enjoying your meal, clean the utensils and bowls promptly to maintain a clean and organized kitchen.

4. Zucchini, Eggplant and Beans Salad

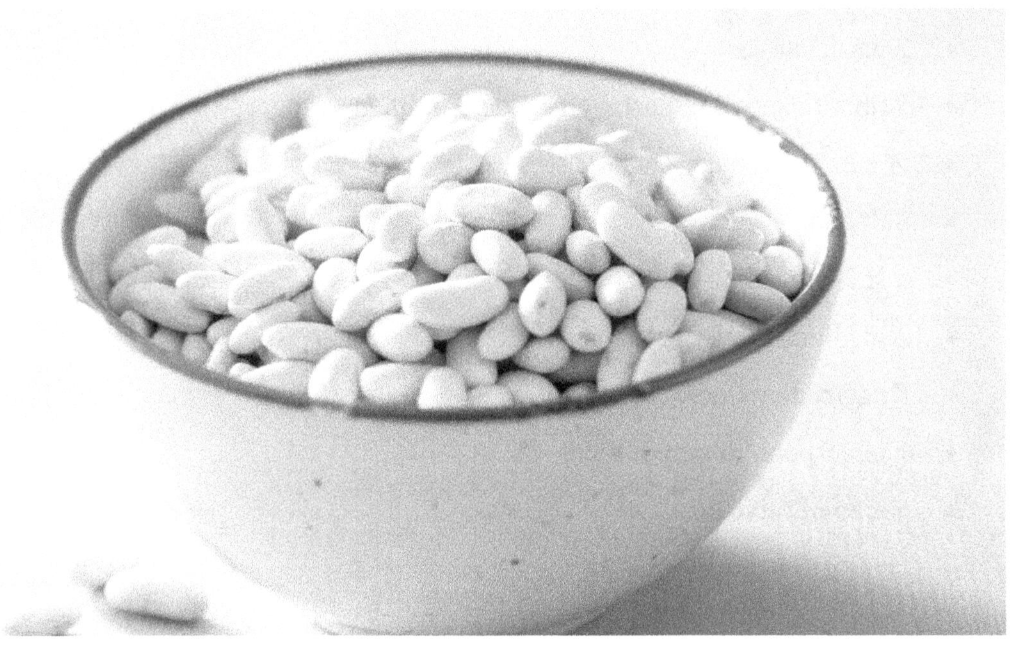

A classic from Mediterranean cuisine, the eggplant is very low in calories and is healthy as it reduces the risk of certain diseases. This salad can be enjoyed hot or cold and if you decide to taste it hot add the beans with the garlic and cumin seeds, and grill the tomatoes too.

Serve: 4

Prep Time: 40 minutes

List of Ingredients:

- 1/3 cup of lemon juice
- 2 garlic cloves
- ¾ lb. of cannellini beans, rinsed and drained
- ½ cup of fresh coriander leaves
- Salt and pepper
- 3 small zucchini
- 2 medium-sized eggplants
- 8 cherry tomatoes, cut in halves
- 1 tablespoon of cumin seeds
- ½ cup of olive oil

sssssssssssssssssss

Methods:

Step 1: Prepare the Vegetables

Begin by cutting the zucchini lengthwise into slices and slicing the eggplant into rounds. The varying shapes add visual appeal and textural variety to the salad.

Step 2: Brush with Olive Oil

Brush all the pieces of zucchini and eggplant with olive oil. This step adds a hint of richness and ensures that the vegetables don't stick to the grill.

Step 3: Grill the Vegetables

Grill the oiled zucchini and eggplant slices until they become browned on both sides and tender. Grilling enhances their natural sweetness and imparts a smoky flavor.

Step 4: Prepare the Seasoned Oil

Warm up the remaining olive oil in a frying pan. This oil will be used to infuse the salad with the flavors of garlic and cumin seeds.

Add minced garlic and cumin seeds to the warm oil. Sauté them for 2 to 3 minutes, allowing their aromas to meld and develop.

Step 5: Assemble the Salad Base

In a large serving bowl, combine the grilled zucchini and eggplant slices. Their charred and tender qualities contribute to the salad's hearty texture.

Step 6: Add Cherry Tomatoes and Beans

Introduce vibrant cherry tomatoes to the bowl, adding a burst of color and refreshing juiciness to the salad.

Add the beans, which offer a satisfying protein and fiber component. You can use canned beans, drained and rinsed, or cook your own from scratch.

Step 7: Infuse with Flavors

Pour the garlic and cumin seed-infused oil over the salad. This seasoned oil adds depth and complexity to the dish, enhancing the overall flavor profile.

Step 8: Add Freshness

Incorporate freshly chopped coriander (also known as cilantro) to the salad. The herb's bright and citrusy notes contrast beautifully with the smoky grilled vegetables.

Step 9: Season and Mix

Drizzle fresh lemon juice over the salad, adding a zesty and tangy element that balances the richness of the grilled vegetables.

Season the salad with salt and pepper to taste, ensuring a well-balanced and harmonious flavor profile.

Step 10: Gently Combine

Gently mix all the ingredients together using a salad server or large spoon. Be careful not to overmix and damage the delicate textures of the ingredients.

Step 11: Present and Serve

Your Zucchini, Eggplant, and Beans Salad is now ready to be enjoyed. The combination of grilled vegetables, beans, and flavorful seasonings makes it a satisfying and nutritious dish.

Fun Facts:

Zucchini and eggplant belong to the same botanical family and are often used interchangeably in Mediterranean dishes.

This salad is not only packed with flavor but also offers a variety of textures from the grilled vegetables and beans.

Cumin seeds are a staple spice in many cuisines and are known for their warm and earthy flavor, as well as potential digestive benefits.

Suggestions:

Elevate the salad's protein content by adding grilled chicken, tofu, or crumbled feta cheese on top.

To make this dish a complete meal, consider serving it over a bed of quinoa, couscous, or mixed greens.

For a nutty crunch and added protein, sprinkle roasted sunflower seeds or chopped almonds over the salad.

Enhance the salad's Mediterranean flair by including sliced Kalamata olives and crumbled feta cheese.

For added complexity, sprinkle some smoked paprika over the salad for a subtle smokiness that complements the grilled vegetables.

To make the salad heartier, mix in cooked quinoa or farro, offering additional protein and fiber.

5. Marinated Sardines with Tomatoes and Raisins

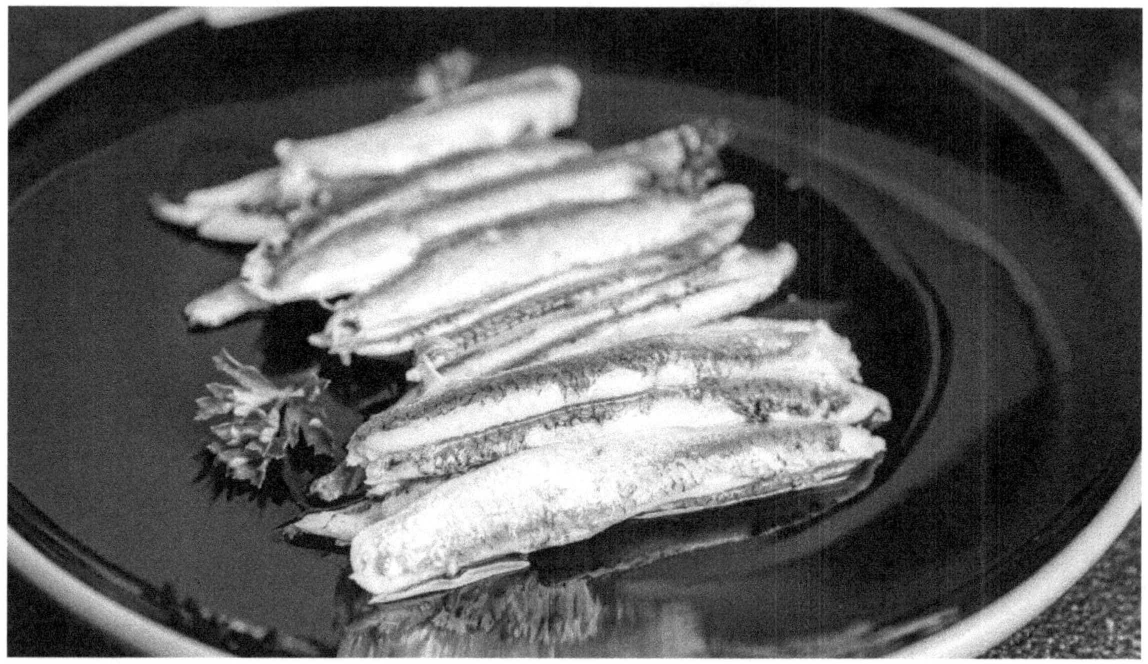

Serve the tasteful appetizer with some crusty bread, so perfect. You can always add some cucumber too. You can also replace the raisins with fresh grapes if the season allows it, which will be even better. Remember, fresh food is always the best.

Serve: 4

Prep Time: 25 minutes

List of Ingredients:

- 1 lemon, juice
- 6 tablespoons of olive oil
- 4 sprigs of fresh thyme
- 3 tablespoons of white wine
- Salt and pepper
- 16 small filets of fresh sardines
- ½ cup of dry raisins
- 6 pitted black olives, cut into halves
- 2 tomatoes

sssssssssssssssssss

Methods:

Step 1: Prepare the Sardines

Begin by cutting the sardine filets into small pieces. This step ensures that the marinated sardines are easy to eat and distribute throughout the dish.

Step 2: Arrange in a Dish

Place the cut sardine pieces in a flat dish. The dish will be used to marinate and infuse the sardines with the flavors of the accompanying ingredients.

Step 3: Mix Olive Oil and Lemon Juice

In a separate bowl, combine the olive oil and lemon juice. The olive oil adds richness and the lemon juice imparts a zesty brightness to the marinade.

Step 4: Enhance the Marinade

Add the raisins and fresh thyme to the olive oil and lemon juice mixture. The raisins provide natural sweetness, and the thyme contributes herbal aromatics to the marinade.

Season the marinade with a pinch of salt and freshly ground black pepper, enhancing the overall flavor profile.

Step 5: Prepare the Tomatoes

Briefly place the tomatoes in boiling water for a few minutes. This step makes it easier to peel the tomatoes and enhances their texture for the marinade.

Step 6: Peel and Crush the Tomatoes

After boiling, drain the tomatoes and peel off their skins. Crush the tomatoes to create a rustic texture that will blend beautifully with the marinade.

Step 7: Incorporate Crushed Tomatoes

Add the crushed tomatoes to the marinade mixture. The combination of fresh tomatoes with the raisins and thyme adds depth and complexity to the flavors.

Step 8: Introduce Olives and White Wine

Add the black olives and a splash of white wine to the marinade mixture. The olives contribute a briny note, while the white wine enhances the marinade's aromatic qualities.

Step 9: Mix and Pour Over Sardines

Mix all the ingredients in the bowl well to ensure even distribution of flavors. Once mixed, pour the marinade over the cut sardines in the dish.

Step 10: Marinate in the Fridge

Cover the dish with the marinating sardines and refrigerate it for at least one hour. This allows the sardines to absorb the flavors and develop a well-rounded taste.

Step 11: Serve and Enjoy

Once marinated, the sardines are ready to be enjoyed. Serve equal portions to everyone and savor the delicious blend of flavors.

Fun Facts:

Sardines are an excellent source of omega-3 fatty acids and provide a range of health benefits, including heart health and brain function.

This dish combines the rich flavors of sardines with the sweet tanginess of tomatoes and raisins, creating a well-balanced and nutritious meal.

Tomatoes are a great source of lycopene, an antioxidant known for its potential health benefits, including reducing the risk of certain chronic diseases.

Suggestions:

For added texture and crunch, sprinkle some toasted pine nuts or slivered almonds over the finished dish.

Serve the marinated sardines on a bed of fresh greens, such as arugula or spinach, for a refreshing contrast.

Experiment with different varieties of tomatoes, such as heirloom or cherry tomatoes, to bring unique flavors and colors to the dish.

For a burst of color and freshness, finely chop some fresh parsley or basil leaves and sprinkle them over the marinated sardines before serving.

Serve the marinated sardines with slices of crusty bread or toasted baguette to sop up the flavorful marinade.

Enhance the dish by adding a sprinkle of crumbled feta cheese over the marinated sardines, offering a creamy and tangy contrast.

For a twist, consider using golden raisins instead of regular raisins. The golden raisins add a touch of sweetness and visual contrast to the dish.

6. Butter Chicken

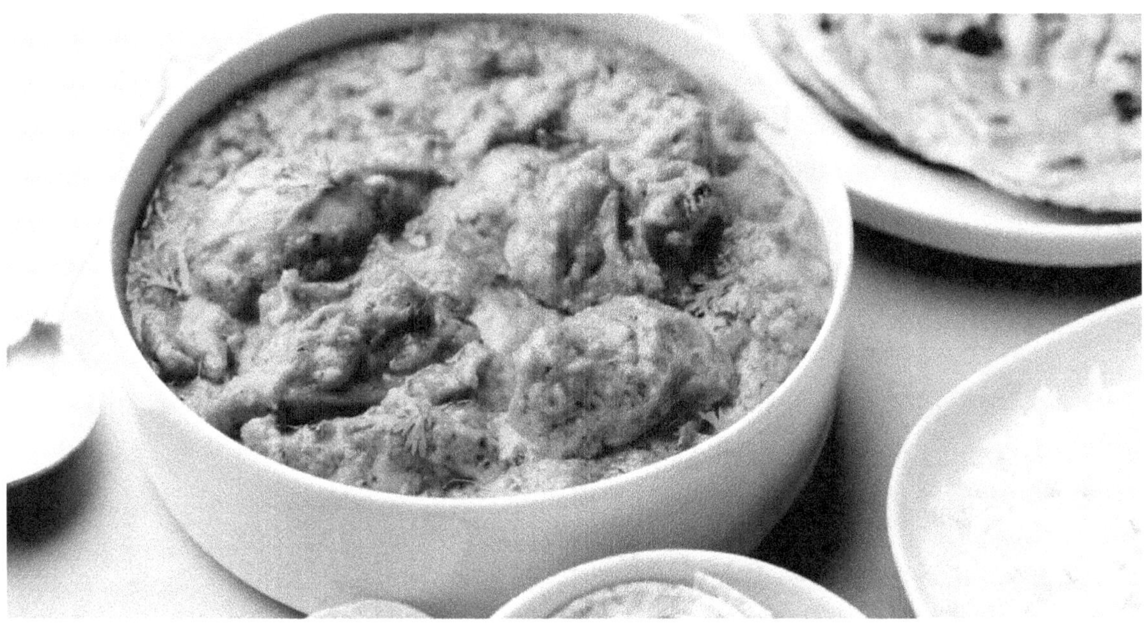

Butter Chicken is a super popular dish in most of the countries in the Middle East and Pakistan. It is also popular as Tikka Masala in India and is made with a yogurt base.

Serve: 4

Prep Time: 1 hour 10 minutes

List of Ingredients:

- 2 tablespoons of garam masala
- 1/4 pound of unsalted butter
- 1-1/2 kg of chicken thighs
- 1/2 cup of fresh cilantro leaves
- 1-1/2 cups of cream
- 3/4 cup of low-sodium chicken stock
- 1 pinch of black pepper
- 2 red seeded sweet pepper, diced
- 2 medium tomatoes, diced
- 1 cinnamon stick
- 4 garlic cloves, minced
- 2 medium onions, peeled and diced
- 2 tablespoons of coconut oil
- 1-1/2 cups of non-fat Greek yogurt
- 1-1/2 tablespoons of ground turmeric
- 2 tablespoons of lemon extract
- 2 tablespoons of ground cumin
- 3 tablespoons of ground almonds
- 2 teaspoons of tomato paste
- 1 pinch of kosher salt
- 1 tablespoon of cumin seeds
- 3 tablespoons of fresh ginger, grated and peeled

sssssssssssssssssss

Methods:

Step 1: Marinate the Chicken

In a mixing bowl, combine cumin, garam masala, lemon juice, and yogurt. This mixture serves as a flavorful marinade for the chicken.

Add the chicken pieces to the marinade, ensuring they are well-coated. Allow the chicken to marinate for 24 hours. Marinating the chicken enhances its flavor and tenderness.

Step 2: Sauté Onions and Aromatics

In a large skillet, melt the butter over medium heat. The butter adds richness to the dish and forms the base of the sauce.

Toss in the sliced onions and sauté for 6-8 minutes until they become soft and translucent. The onions provide a sweet and savory flavor to the sauce.

Step 3: Add Aromatics

To the sautéed onions, add cumin seeds, grated ginger, and minced garlic. These aromatic ingredients infuse the dish with a fragrant and distinctive taste.

Continue cooking until the onions caramelize and the aromatics release their flavors.

Step 4: Cook the Marinated Chicken

Add the marinated chicken to the skillet, including the marinade. Cook the chicken for about 5 minutes, stirring occasionally to ensure even cooking.

Cooking the chicken in the aromatic base allows it to absorb the flavors of the spices and onions.

Step 5: Simmer with Chicken Stock

Pour chicken stock into the skillet and bring the mixture to a simmer. Allow it to simmer for half an hour, ensuring the chicken cooks through and the flavors meld together.

Keep the pan uncovered to allow the sauce to thicken and develop its richness.

Step 6: Creamy Tomato Base

Stir in tomato paste and cream to the simmering chicken mixture. The tomato paste adds a tangy and vibrant flavor, while the cream creates a luscious and velvety texture.

Cook the mixture over low heat for an additional 15 minutes, allowing the flavors to meld and the sauce to thicken.

Step 7: Final Touches

Remove the skillet from the heat and toss in slivered almonds and fresh cilantro leaves. These additions provide crunch and freshness to the dish, enhancing its overall texture and flavor.

Cover the pan and let it rest for 5 minutes before serving. This resting period allows the flavors to meld and intensify.

Step 8: Serve and Savor

Spoon the flavorful butter chicken over a bed of rice or alongside naan bread. Garnish with extra cilantro leaves if desired.

Fun Facts:

Butter chicken, also known as "Murgh Makhani," is a popular Indian dish known for its rich and creamy tomato-based sauce.

The dish is believed to have originated in the Punjabi region of India and has gained worldwide popularity due to its flavorful and comforting taste.

Butter chicken is often enjoyed with a side of naan bread or rice to soak up the delicious sauce.

Suggestions:

Serve butter chicken with naan bread or fragrant basmati rice for a complete and satisfying meal.

Customize the level of spiciness by adjusting the amount of garam masala and red chili powder to suit your taste preferences.

For a lighter version, use Greek yogurt instead of heavy cream to achieve a creamy consistency with fewer calories.

Serve butter chicken with a cooling cucumber raita or a side of pickled vegetables to balance out the richness of the dish.

Elevate your meal by making homemade naan bread to complement the butter chicken. The soft and pillowy naan is perfect for scooping up the flavorful sauce.

Customize the level of spiciness by adjusting the amount of red chili powder in the marinade and sauce. Add more or less based on your preference for heat.

Embrace the culinary journey by learning more about the history and cultural significance of butter chicken in Indian cuisine.

7. Spicy and Sweet Pad Thai

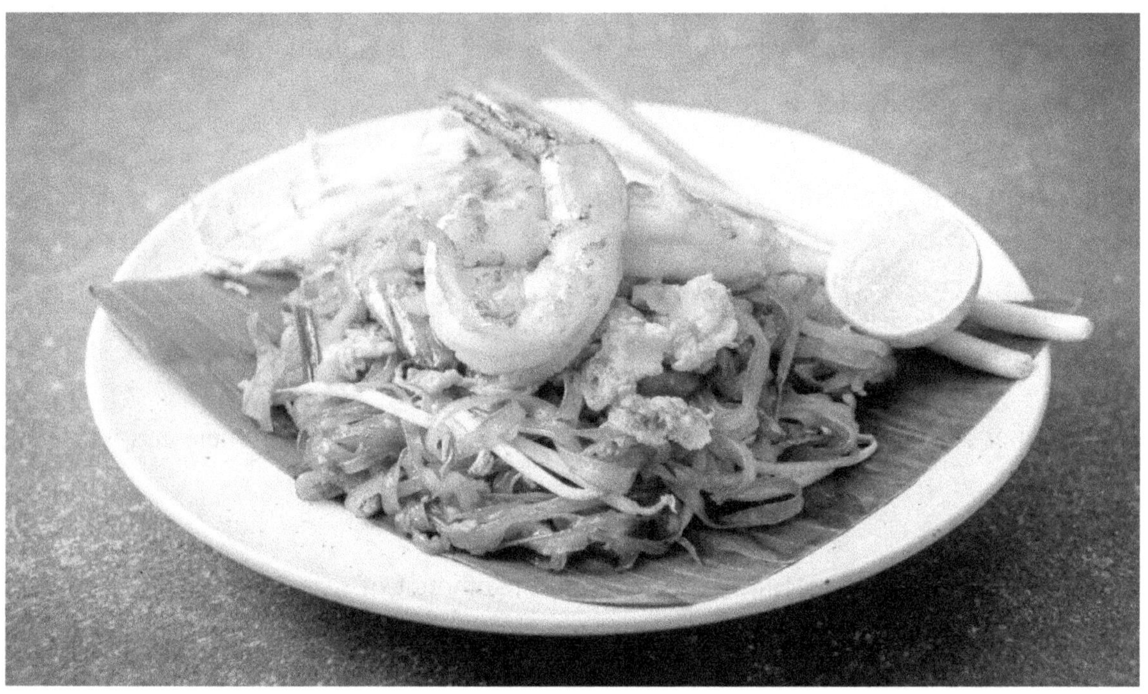

Pad Thai is a very popular dish in Thailand. It is made with rice noodles, vegetables and chicken or seafood. This dish can be enjoyed with extra side dishes or served up as leftovers for lunch the next day.

Serve: 5

Prep Time: 35 minutes

List of Ingredients:

- 2 tablespoons of fresh cilantro leaves
- 1/2 cup of shredded carrots
- 1/2 cup of chopped peanuts
- 1 pinch of ground red pepper
- 1/4 cup of lemon extract or lime juice
- 1 package of Thai rice noodles
- 1 package of tofu, cubed
- 1 tablespoon of peanut oil
- 2 garlic cloves, finely minced
- 1 sweet red pepper, seeded and minced
- 1 tablespoon of honey
- 1/4 cup of soy sauce
- 1/2 cup of sliced mushrooms

sssssssssssssssssss

Methods:

Step 1: Sautéing the Veggies

Heat oil in a saucepan over medium heat.

Add tofu, sliced mushrooms, bell peppers, and minced garlic to the pan.

Cook until the vegetables soften and the tofu begins to brown, creating a delicious base of flavors.

Step 2: Cooking the Noodles

Boil the noodles in a separate pot for 15-20 minutes, or until they reach your desired level of tenderness.

Drain the noodles and set them aside for later use.

Step 3: Creating the Flavorful Sauce

In a bowl, combine crushed red pepper, honey (for sweetness), soy sauce (for savory umami), and freshly squeezed lime juice (for tanginess).

Mix these ingredients to create a balanced sauce that captures the essence of Pad Thai's signature flavors.

Step 4: Sauce Infusion

Pour the prepared sauce mixture over the cooked vegetables in the saucepan.

Gently stir and let the flavors meld together as the mixture simmers.

After about 5 minutes, remove the pan from the heat. The sauce will coat the veggies with its spicy and sweet profile.

Step 5: Assembling the Dish

Divide the cooked noodles into individual serving bowls, creating a base for the Pad Thai.

Top each bowl with fresh cilantro leaves, shredded carrots, and chopped peanuts. These additions contribute to the dish's vibrant colors and textures.

Step 6: Pouring the Broth

Carefully ladle the flavorful broth from the saucepan into each serving bowl, ensuring that the noodles and toppings are well coated.

Step 7: Serve and Enjoy

Your spicy and sweet Pad Thai is now ready to be savored.

Serve the bowls while they're still hot to fully appreciate the melding of flavors.

Fun Facts:

Pad Thai is a popular Thai street food dish known for its blend of spicy, sweet, and savory flavors.

This recipe offers a homemade version of Pad Thai that combines a variety of colorful vegetables, protein-rich tofu, and a tantalizing sauce.

The combination of honey and lime juice in the sauce adds a unique contrast of flavors, enhancing both the sweetness and tanginess of the dish.

Suggestions:

Customize the level of spiciness by adjusting the amount of crushed red pepper to suit your taste preferences.

Experiment with protein options such as shrimp, chicken, or tempeh for a twist on the classic recipe.

Garnish the bowls with extra cilantro leaves, lime wedges, and a sprinkle of sesame seeds for an attractive presentation.

Enjoy your Pad Thai alongside a refreshing Thai iced tea or a citrus-infused sparkling water for a well-balanced meal.

If you have leftovers, store them in an airtight container in the refrigerator. Reheat gently on the stovetop or in the microwave.

Host a Pad Thai night with friends and family, encouraging everyone to customize their bowls with additional toppings like bean sprouts, lime wedges, and fresh herbs.

Experiment with different types of noodles, such as rice noodles, egg noodles, or even zucchini noodles (zoodles) for a low-carb option.

Combine elements from other cuisines by adding ingredients like sliced avocado, chopped mango, or even grilled pineapple for a creative fusion twist on traditional Pad Thai.

8. Crab Salad with Tomato Dressing

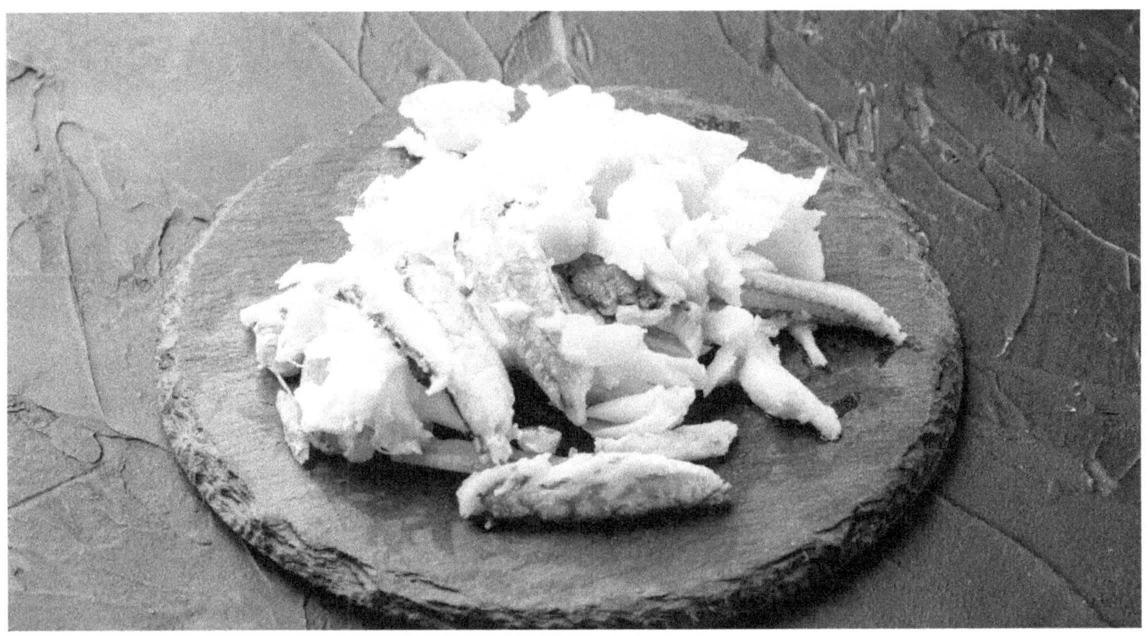

This chubby bulb vegetable is full of water and valuable minerals, including potassium and magnesium. The calcium is also very high. It displays a level of iron well above the average and is a champion of Vitamin C, E, and B9. So, don't wait and eat some fennel, get used to it and enjoy it.

Serve: 4

Prep Time: 35 minutes

List of Ingredients:

- 2 tablespoons of tomato juice
- 5 tablespoons of olive oil
- 1 teaspoon of tarragon
- ½ cucumber, cut into very small diced
- A dash of Worcester sauce
- 1 tablespoon of balsamic vinegar
- 9 oz. of fresh crab or canned crab meat
- 1 large bulb of fennel, thinly sliced
- 3 oz. of mixed salad leaves
- 1 tablespoon of chives
- 1 tablespoon of paprika
- 2 large tomatoes

ssssssssssssssssss

Methods:

Step 1: Preparing the Tomatoes

Place the tomatoes in a bowl and pour hot water over them. Let them sit for about 30 seconds. This process makes it easier to peel the tomatoes.

Step 2: Dicing the Tomatoes

Remove the skin from the tomatoes and deseed them. Dice the tomatoes into small pieces, ensuring you collect and keep the juice that comes out during the process.

Step 3: Making the Tomato Dressing

Whisk together the olive oil and balsamic vinegar in a small bowl. The combination of these ingredients will create a flavorful and tangy dressing.

Add the freshly chopped tarragon and a dash of Worcester sauce to the dressing for added depth of flavor.

Incorporate the collected tomato juice from dicing the tomatoes into the dressing. This will infuse the dressing with the natural sweetness and aroma of the tomatoes. Season the dressing to taste.

Step 4: Preparing the Crab Salad

In a large bowl, combine the crab meat and finely sliced fennel. The fennel adds a subtle crunch and a hint of anise flavor that compliments the crab.

Dice the cucumber and add it to the bowl with the crab and fennel. The cucumber provides a refreshing contrast to the richness of the crab meat.

Step 5: Mixing the Salad

Gently mix the diced tomatoes into the crab salad. The tomatoes add juiciness and vibrant color to the dish.

Step 6: Adding the Tomato Dressing

Pour the prepared tomato dressing over the crab salad mixture. The dressing will coat the ingredients, enhancing the overall flavor profile of the salad.

Step 7: Incorporating the Dressing

Thoroughly mix the crab salad with the tomato dressing to ensure that all the ingredients are well coated.

Step 8: Serving the Crab Salad

Arrange a bed of mixed salad leaves on serving plates.

Portion the crab salad with tomato dressing onto each plate. The vibrant colors and enticing aromas will make it an appealing dish.

Step 9: Enjoying the Freshness

Delight in the fresh combination of crab, tomatoes, and cucumber in every bite. The tomato dressing brings all the flavors together harmoniously.

Fun Facts:

This crab salad combines the freshness of tomatoes and cucumbers with the delicate flavor of crab meat, creating a light and flavorful dish.

Tomatoes provide a burst of color, nutrients, and a refreshing taste to the salad.

Suggestions:

Serve this crab salad as a refreshing appetizer or a light main course during a sunny outdoor gathering.

Pair the salad with a crisp white wine to complement the seafood and bright flavors.

For an elegant touch, garnish the crab salad with a sprig of fresh tarragon or a sprinkle of chopped parsley.

Consider serving the crab salad with crusty bread or a light citrus vinaigrette for an additional layer of flavor.

Explore variations of the crab salad by adding ingredients like avocado slices, toasted nuts, or a squeeze of lemon juice to create your unique twist.

Take a moment to savor the delicate flavors of the crab meat, perfectly complemented by the bright and tangy tomato dressing.

9. Quinoa Lentil Salad

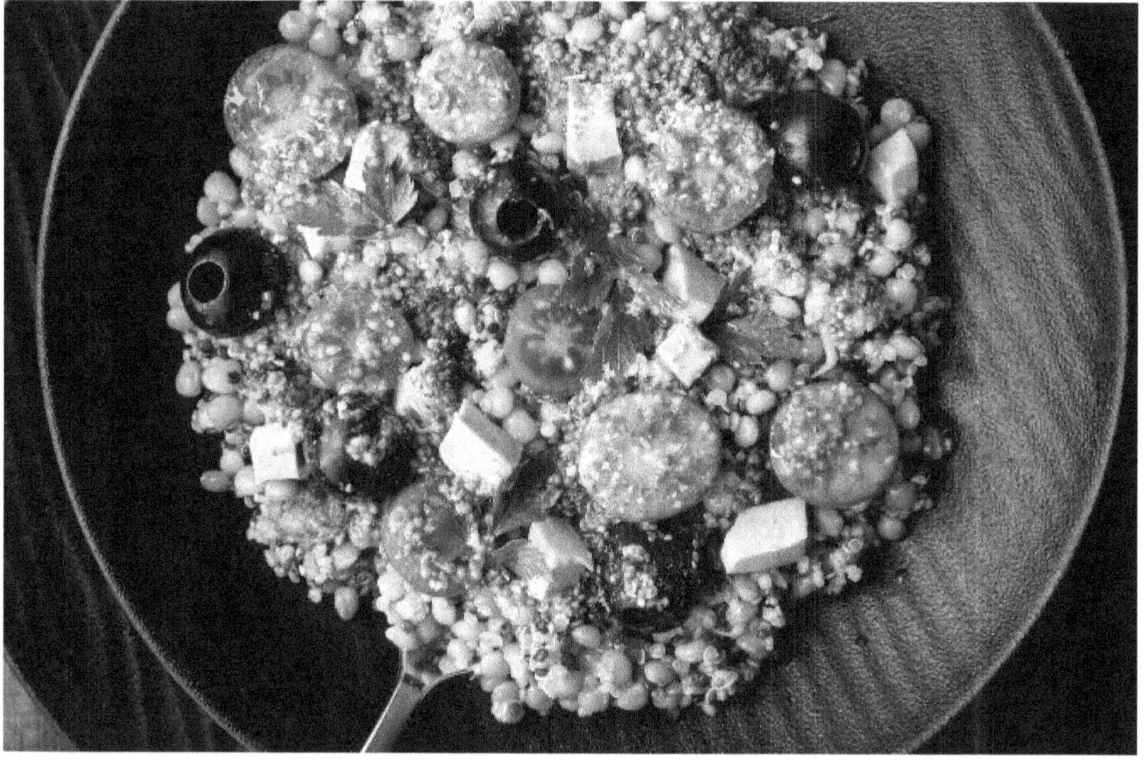

Lentils are another great source of protein that is very good for you. They can be used in many different ways to create a salad or even a soup. Quinoa can be used as a cereal or even as a side dish with vegetables.

Serve: 4

Prep Time: 25 minutes

List of Ingredients:

- 1 yellow sweet pepper, diced
- 1 shallot, chopped
- 2 teaspoons of Dijon mustard
- 1/4 cup of lemon juice
- 1/3 cup of crumbled feta cheese
- 1 pinch of salt
- 2/3 cup of dried brown lentils
- 2 cups of water
- 1 cup of quinoa
- 1 bunch of arugula, finely chopped
- 1/4 cup of extra virgin olive oil
- 4 tablespoons of fresh mint, chopped

sssssssssssssssssss

Methods:

Step 1: Boiling the Saltwater

In a saucepan, bring 2 cups of saltwater to a vigorous boil. This saltwater infusion will contribute flavor and seasoning to both the lentils and quinoa, enhancing the overall taste of the salad.

Step 2: Veggie Immersion

Gently introduce an array of colorful vegetables into the bubbling saltwater. Allow them to bask in the heat, cooking gently for a duration of 30 minutes. This simmering process ensures that the vegetables absorb the saltwater's essence while maintaining their vibrant colors and crisp textures.

Step 3: Lentil Preparation

Once the lentils have undergone their savory bath, drain them, bidding farewell to the infused water. Set the now-seasoned vegetables aside as well, preserving their cooked integrity.

Step 4: Quinoa Elevation

Embark on a culinary journey by boiling yet another batch of saltwater. This time, the quinoa takes center stage. Cook the quinoa in the simmering pan of saltwater until it achieves a fluffy and slightly translucent texture. This step introduces a nutty and wholesome component to your salad.

Step 5: Tangy Fusion

In a separate bowl, combine freshly ground pepper, a pinch of salt, zesty mustard, invigorating lemon juice, and a drizzle of oil. Mix these elements together to form a harmonious and tangy dressing that will enrobe your salad with flavor.

Step 6: Assembling the Ensemble

Invite the cooked vegetables to gather in a larger bowl, awaiting the flavorful embrace of the tangy dressing. Once the vegetables are nestled in their new abode, pour the prepared dressing over them, ensuring every morsel is kissed by its zesty goodness.

Step 7: Minty Zest and Feta Finesse

Sprinkle the vibrancy of fresh mint leaves over the vegetable ensemble, imparting a refreshing burst of herbaceous flavor. Elevate the dish further by generously scattering crumbled feta cheese over the salad, adding a delightful creaminess and a hint of saltiness.

Step 8: Savory Celebration

Your Quinoa Lentil Salad is now ready to be enjoyed. Serve this nutrient-packed creation to your taste buds' delight, savoring the harmony of textures, flavors, and colors that dance within each mouthful.

Fun Facts:

Quinoa and lentils are both excellent sources of plant-based protein, making this salad a nutritious and filling option.

The combination of fresh vegetables, quinoa, and lentils creates a colorful and vibrant dish that's as visually appealing as it is delicious.

Did you know? Mint not only adds a burst of freshness but also offers potential digestive benefits.

Suggestions:

Customize your Quinoa Lentil Salad by adding your favorite vegetables and herbs. Try cucumbers, bell peppers, or cherry tomatoes for added crunch and flavor.

To enhance the Mediterranean flair, consider adding Kalamata olives and a sprinkle of chopped parsley to the salad.

10. Salmon Salad

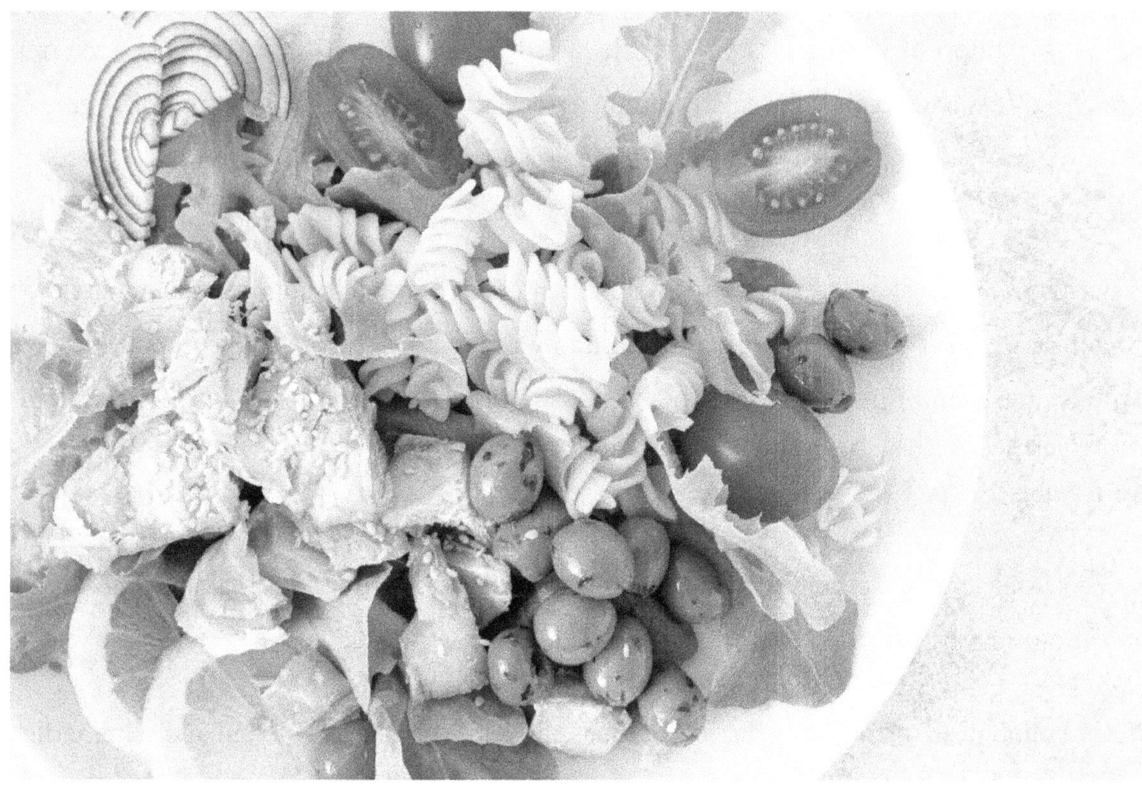

Salmon and veggies on a bed of lettuce. This is a very delicious combination. You can make it as spicy or as bland as you want.

Serve: 4

Prep Time: 45 minutes

List of Ingredients:

- 1 tablespoon of fresh dill, finely chopped
- 1 tablespoon of extra-virgin olive oil
- 1/4 teaspoon of freshly ground pepper
- A pinch of salt
- 2 large filets of wild salmon, either poached or grilled and then chilled
- 1 cup of cherry tomatoes, halved
- 2 red onions, sliced
- 1 tablespoon of balsamic vinegar
- 1 tablespoon of capers

sssssssssssssssssss

Methods:

Step 1: Salmon Prep

Begin by removing the skin and bones from the poached or grilled salmon filets. This step ensures that your salmon is ready to be transformed into delectable chunks that will form the foundation of your salad.

Step 2: Chunk Creation

Break the cooled salmon into bite-sized chunks and place them in a bowl. The chunks should be large enough to retain their texture while blending harmoniously with the other ingredients.

Step 3: Ingredient Ensemble

Introduce the halved cherry tomatoes, sliced red onion, and capers into the bowl with the salmon. Gently toss these ingredients together, allowing them to mingle and create a colorful and flavorful medley.

Step 4: Flavorful Fusion

In a separate bowl, create a delightful dressing by combining extra-virgin olive oil, balsamic vinegar, and finely chopped fresh dill. This dressing infuses the salad with a blend of tangy, herbal, and rich flavors that complement the salmon.

Step 5: Dressing Embrace

Pour the olive oil, balsamic vinegar, and dill mixture over the salmon chunks and the accompanying ingredients. Toss the components once more, ensuring that the dressing coats each element evenly, uniting the flavors in a harmonious blend.

Step 6: Seasonal Symphony

Elevate the flavors of your salmon salad by sprinkling a pinch of salt and freshly ground pepper over the ensemble. Adjust the seasoning to your taste preferences, allowing the salt and pepper to amplify the flavors without overpowering them.

Step 7: Chilling Elegance

Let your salmon salad rest in the refrigerator for at least half an hour before serving. This chilling period not only allows the flavors to meld and intensify but also ensures that the salad is served at an invitingly cool temperature.

Fun Facts:

Salmon is a nutritional powerhouse, rich in omega-3 fatty acids that are beneficial for heart and brain health.

Dill not only adds a fresh and herby flavor but also provides potential digestive and antioxidant benefits to the salad.

Did you know? Balsamic vinegar's sweet and tangy profile complements the richness of salmon, creating a delightful contrast of flavors.

Suggestions:

Customize your salmon salad by adding ingredients like avocado slices, cucumber, or mixed greens for added freshness and texture.

Serve the chilled salmon salad on a bed of mixed greens or as a filling for whole-grain wraps for a well-rounded meal.

11. Lentils and Bulgur Rosti with Yogurt Dressing

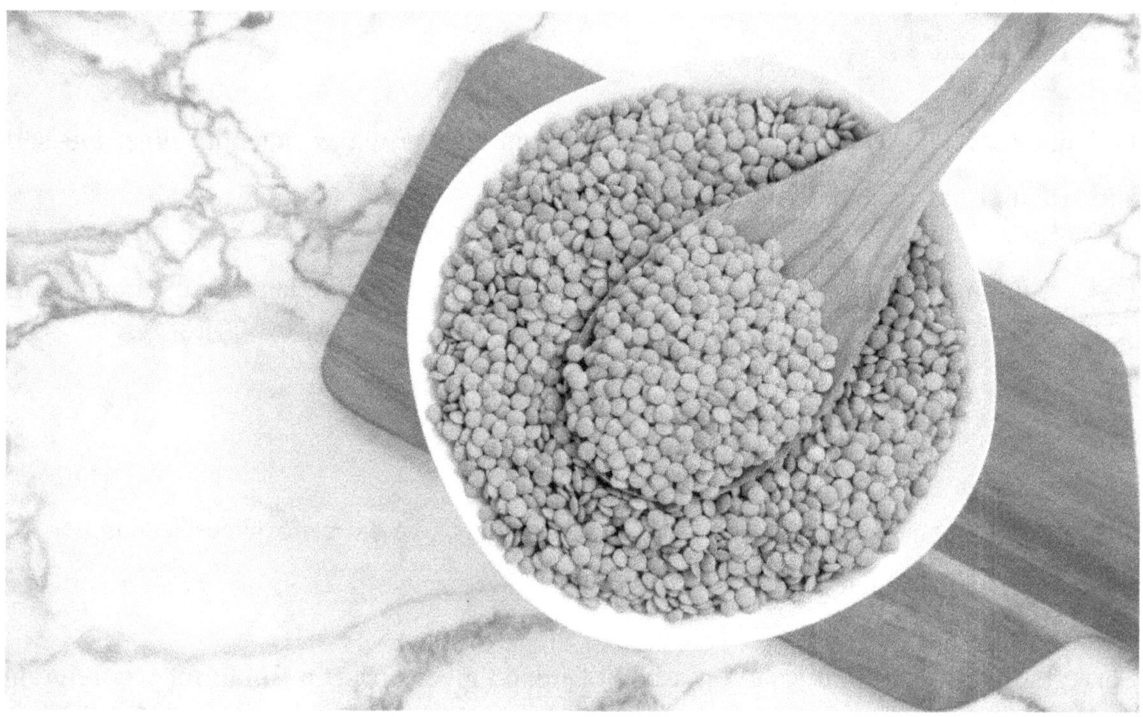

Rosti can be made with all sorts of different List of Ingredients and not always potatoes. Make it as thick as you want, obviously the thicker you do, the longer it needs to cook on each side. If you cannot find some bulgur, use another cereal.

Serve: 4

Prep Time: 1 hour 10 minutes

List of Ingredients:

- 1 onion, finely chopped
- 3 tablespoons of fresh mints
- 4 eggs, beaten
- ½ cup of flour
- 1 garlic clove, thinly chopped
- Salt and pepper
- 1/3 lb. of lentils
- ¼ lb. of bulgur
- 5 tablespoons of olive oil
- 3 teaspoons of cumin
- 2 teaspoons of powder coriander
- 1 small cucumber, cut into very small cubes
- ½ cup of yogurt

sssssssssssssssssss

Methods:

Step 1: Lentil Boil

Begin by heating a pan of water until it reaches a boiling point. Once the water is boiling, add the lentils to the pan and allow them to cook for approximately 30 minutes or until they achieve a tender consistency. This step lays the foundation for the lentil component of your rosti.

Step 2: Water Balance

Once the lentils are cooked, ensure that there is just enough water to cover them. This step involves stopping the cooking process and adjusting the water level to create the ideal base for the rosti.

Step 3: Bulgur Integration

Add the bulgur to the pan with the lentils, creating a harmonious blend of ingredients. Leave this mixture on the side to rest and meld flavors for at least 1 hour and 30 minutes. This resting period allows the bulgur to absorb the flavors and moisture from the lentils.

Step 4: Yogurt Dressing

While the lentil and bulgur mixture rests, prepare the yogurt dressing. Mix yogurt with finely minced garlic and cucumber in a bowl. This refreshing dressing will complement the earthy flavors of the rosti.

Step 5: Flavorful Composition

After the resting period, introduce diced onion, cumin, mint, coriander, eggs, and flour to the lentil and bulgur mixture in the pan. Blend all these ingredients together until they form a cohesive and compact composition, ready to be transformed into delicious rosti.

Step 6: Rosti Formation

Warm up olive oil in a large frying pan over medium heat. Use a large spoon to place portions of the compact mixture in the pan, forming individual rosti. Cook each side until they achieve a golden brown hue, approximately 2 minutes on each side. Repeat this process until you've used all of the mixture to create a delightful batch of rosti.

Step 7: Serving Elegance

Arrange the cooked rosti on serving plates. Accompany each serving with a generous dollop of the prepared yogurt dressing, allowing the creamy and tangy flavors to complement the warm and crispy rosti.

Fun Facts:

Lentils are a fantastic source of plant-based protein and dietary fiber, making this dish both nutritious and satisfying.

Bulgur adds a nutty and chewy texture to the rosti, enhancing the overall eating experience.

Did you know? Yogurt dressing not only complements the flavors but also offers a cooling contrast to the warm and crispy rosti.

Suggestions:

Garnish your lentil and bulgur rosti with a sprinkle of chopped fresh herbs, such as parsley or chives, for added color and freshness.

Enjoy these rosti as a main dish or serve them as a side to grilled vegetables or a crisp salad for a well-rounded meal.

12. Chicken Casserole

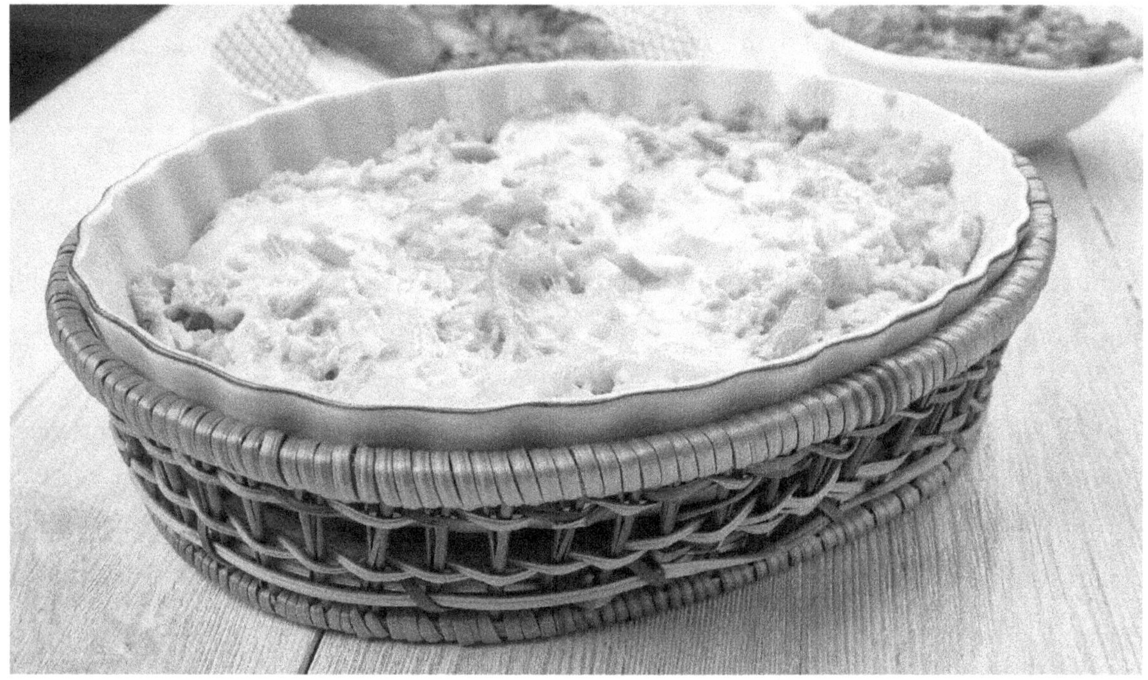

The chicken can be prepared and enjoyed in thousands of different ways. But sometimes, it is industrially deformed to the point that only the word "chicken" on the packaging enables us to know what it is … it's a shame! So give yourself the pleasure of a real chicken and enjoy without excess.

Serve: 4

Prep Time: 1 hour 10 minutes

List of Ingredients:

- 4 large potatoes, cut into four pieces each of them
- ½ cup of white wine
- 1 onion, chopped
- 6 oz. of black olives, stoned
- 1 tablespoon of thyme
- 1 bay leaf
- Salt and pepper
- 1 whole chicken, cut into 8 pieces
- 2 garlic cloves, crushed
- 2 tablespoons of olive oil
- 1 green and red peppers, cut in strips
- 1 large canned of chopped tomatoes

sssssssssssssssssss

Methods:

Step 1: Olive Oil Prelude

Begin by warming olive oil in a large saucepan over medium heat. This initial step sets the foundation for the flavors to come and provides a canvas for the casserole's elements.

Step 2: Chicken Sear

Introduce the chicken pieces to the warmed olive oil and sauté them until they achieve a delectable golden brown hue on all sides. The process of browning the chicken enhances its flavor and contributes to the overall richness of the casserole.

Step 3: Chicken Pause

Once the chicken pieces have achieved the desired color, carefully remove them from the pan and set them aside. This brief pause allows the chicken to rest while you move on to the next steps.

Step 4: Aromatics Introduce

Add the diced onion and minced garlic to the pan, creating a fragrant foundation for the casserole. Sauté these aromatics until they become tender and release their enticing scents.

Step 5: Pepper and Tomato Medley

Introduce the green and red bell peppers, along with the tomatoes, to the sautéed onion and garlic. This colorful medley of vegetables adds vibrancy and texture to the casserole, infusing it with a spectrum of flavors.

Step 6: Chicken Reunion

Reintroduce the golden-brown chicken pieces back into the pan. This step allows the chicken to reunite with the aromatic vegetable mixture, setting the stage for a harmonious fusion of flavors.

Step 7: Wine and Herbs Elegance

Pour in the white wine, infusing the casserole with a sophisticated layer of flavor. Add the thyme, bay leaf, black olives, and potatoes. Season the mixture, creating a symphony of taste that's both comforting and inviting.

Step 8: Simmer Symphony

Bring the casserole to a gentle boil before reducing the heat to low. Allow the flavors to meld and intensify as the casserole simmers for a leisurely 45 minutes. Stir the mixture occasionally to ensure even cooking and flavor distribution.

Step 9: Culinary Crescendo

As the 45-minute simmering period concludes, the chicken casserole is now at its flavorful peak. Serve the hearty and aromatic dish immediately, savoring the rich blend of textures and tastes that this creation offers.

Fun Facts:

Casseroles are known for their comfort and versatility, often incorporating a medley of flavors and textures in a single dish.

Thyme and bay leaf lend aromatic depth to the casserole, enhancing the overall taste experience.

Did you know? Casseroles often taste even better the next day as the flavors continue to meld and intensify upon reheating.

Suggestions:

Customize your chicken casserole by adding vegetables like carrots, zucchini, or mushrooms for additional color and nutrients.

Serve the casserole with a side of crusty bread or fluffy rice to soak up the flavorful sauce.

13. Smoked Chicken Salad

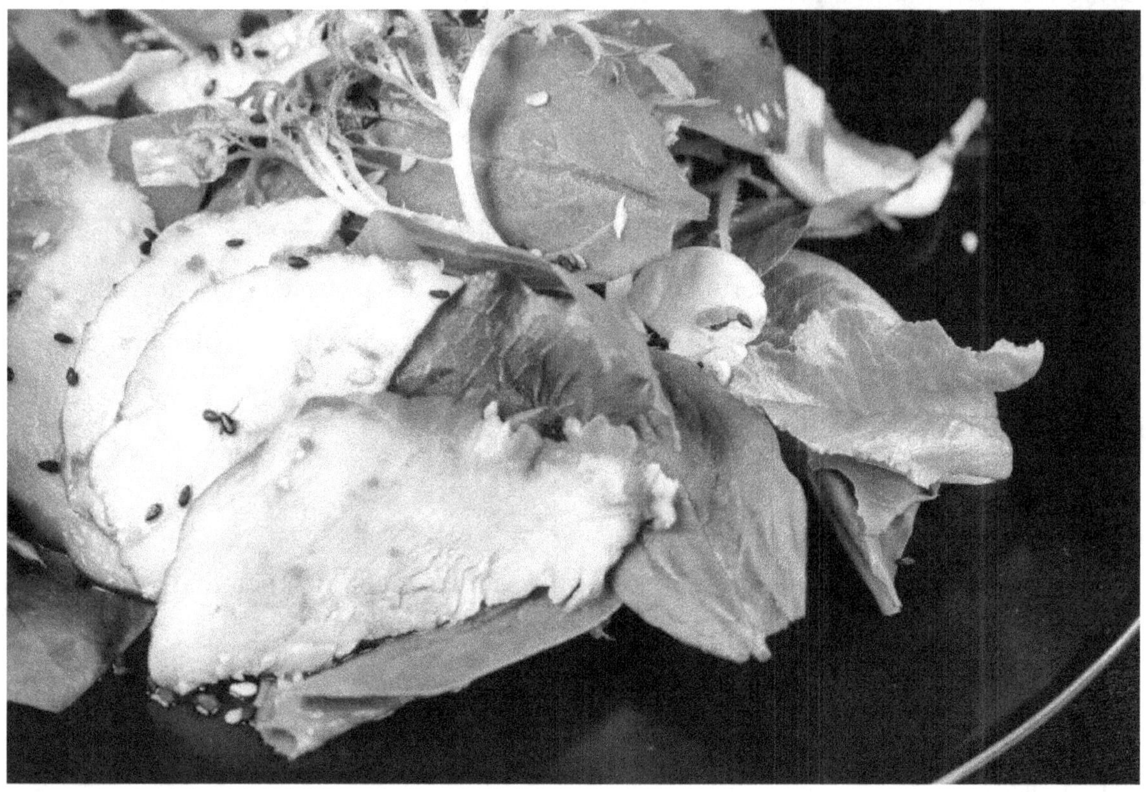

Smoked chicken has already been cooked during the curing process, making this a simple salad to throw together at short notice. You can keep the smoked chicken in the freezer. Try to use a local natural honey without any other things added to it.

Serve: 4

Prep Time: 15 minutes

List of Ingredients:

- 1 cup of basil leaves
- ¼ cup of lime juice
- 1 tablespoon of honey
- 1 small red chili, seeded, chopped finely
- 2 tablespoons of olive oil
- Salt and pepper
- ½ lb. of baby spinach leaves
- 1 oak leaf salad
- 7/8 lb. of smoked chicken breast, sliced
- 1 yellow pepper
- 1 red onion

sssssssssssssssssss

Methods:

Step 1: Fresh Greens Preparations

Begin by washing and draining the oak leaf and baby spinach leaves. This step ensures that the greens are clean and ready to be used as the base of the salad.

Step 2: Salad Assembly

Combine the washed oak leaf and baby spinach leaves in a large serving bowl. Gently mix them together to create a harmonious blend of textures and flavors, setting the stage for the remaining ingredients.

Step 3: Vegetable Slicing

Thinly slice the yellow pepper and red onion, creating delicate and colorful additions to the salad. These vibrant vegetables contribute to the salad's visual appeal and offer a delightful crunch.

Step 4: Herb Inclusion

Add fresh basil leaves to the salad, introducing a fragrant and aromatic element that complements the other ingredients. Mixing the basil with the greens adds an herbal note to the overall taste profile.

Step 5: Smoky Chicken Addition

Introduce the smoked chicken to the salad, adding a layer of smokiness and protein. The tender chicken pairs beautifully with the assortment of vegetables and greens.

Step 6: Dressing Harmony

In a small bowl, create the dressing by combining olive oil and lime juice. Add honey and red chili for a balanced blend of flavors. Season the mixture with a touch of salt and pepper, ensuring a harmonious dressing.

Step 7: Dressing Fusion

Whisk the dressing ingredients thoroughly until they combine into a cohesive and flavorful mixture. This dressing will serve as the bridge that brings the different components of the salad together.

Step 8: Dressing Integration

Drizzle the prepared dressing over the salad, ensuring that all the ingredients are evenly coated. Mixing the dressing with the salad ingredients allows each bite to be infused with a symphony of flavors.

Step 9: Culinary Presentation

Your smoked chicken salad is now complete and ready to be served. The array of colors, textures, and flavors offers a delightful dining experience that's both satisfying and nourishing.

Fun Facts:

Smoked chicken adds a distinct and smoky flavor to the salad, enhancing its overall taste.

The combination of different vegetables and herbs provides a variety of textures and colors, making the salad visually appealing.

Did you know? Oak leaf lettuce is known for its tender and delicate leaves, while baby spinach is rich in nutrients and adds a fresh touch to the salad.

Suggestions:

Enhance the salad's protein content by adding nuts, seeds, or boiled eggs as optional toppings.

For added crunch, consider including croutons or toasted pumpkin seeds to complement the salad's textures.

14. Fish Filets with Its Little Vegetables

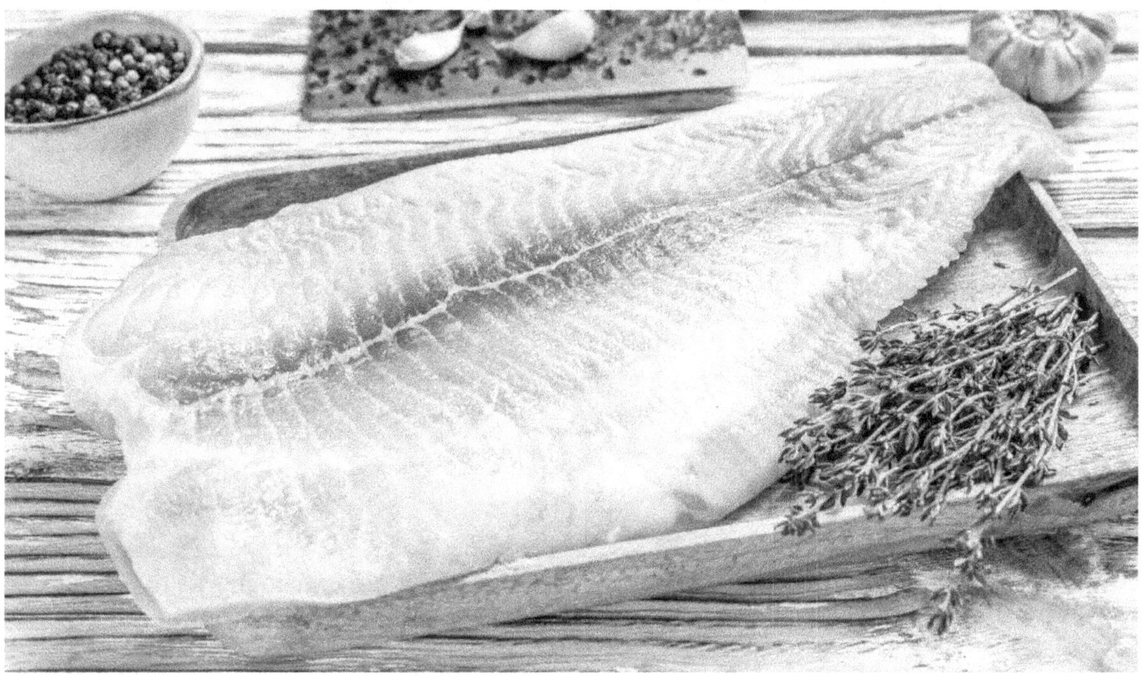

Full flavor is on; your taste buds will be delighted by this smooth taste. Don't hesitate to add other vegetables if you want and if you do, please, adjust the quantity of liquid too. Serve it with a mixed salad or even a nice homemade mashed potato.

Serve: 4

Prep Time: 40 minutes

List of Ingredients:

- 1 glass of white wine
- 3 tablespoons of single cream
- 1 teaspoon of thyme
- Salt and pepper
- 4 filets of white fish, like cod, etc.
- 1 leek, finely sliced
- 2 carrots, finely sliced
- 1 shallot, chopped
- 1 tablespoon of olive oil

sssssssssssssssssss

Methods:

Step 1: Oven Preheating

Begin by preheating the oven to 350°F (175°C). This ensures that the oven is at the ideal temperature for baking the fish filets and vegetables.

Step 2: Frying Pan Warming

Heat olive oil in a frying pan over medium heat. The olive oil serves as the base for sautéing the shallot and vegetables, infusing them with flavor.

Step 3: Shallot Sautéing

Add the finely chopped shallot to the heated oil in the frying pan. Sauté the shallot until it becomes tender and aromatic, releasing its flavors into the oil.

Step 4: Vegetable Combination

Introduce the sliced leeks and carrots to the sautéed shallot in the pan. Cook the vegetables over low heat for approximately 5 minutes. Stir occasionally to ensure even cooking and prevent sticking.

Step 5: Wine Infusion

Pour white wine into the pan with the cooked vegetables. Allow the wine to simmer and reduce for an additional 5 minutes, imparting its subtle flavors to the vegetable mixture.

Step 6: Creamy Harmony

Pour cream into the pan with the vegetables and wine reduction. Season the mixture with desired seasonings to enhance the flavors. The cream adds richness to the dish's sauce.

Step 7: Oven Dish Assembly

Place the fish filets in individual oven-safe dishes. The fish filets will serve as the base for the flavorful vegetable mixture.

Step 8: Vegetable Blanket

Cover the fish filets with the cooked vegetable mixture, creating a comforting and flavorful "blanket" of leeks, carrots, and shallots over the fish.

Step 9: Thyme Sprinkling

Sprinkle fresh or dried thyme leaves over the top of the assembled fish and vegetable dishes. Thyme's earthy aroma enhances the overall dish with its aromatic qualities.

Step 10: Baking Brilliance

Bake the assembled dishes in the preheated oven for approximately 15 to 20 minutes. This baking duration ensures that the fish filets are cooked to perfection and the flavors meld together.

Step 11: Culinary Enjoyment

Once baked, remove the fish filets with their accompanying vegetables from the oven. The dish is now ready to be served, offering a harmonious blend of fish, vegetables, and a creamy sauce.

Fun Facts:

This dish combines tender fish filets with a medley of vegetables, resulting in a delightful and balanced meal.

The addition of white wine and cream imparts a rich and flavorful sauce that complements the fish and vegetables.

Did you know? Leeks belong to the same family as onions and garlic and add a mild and slightly sweet flavor to the dish.

Suggestions:

Opt for a white fish variety such as cod, haddock, or tilapia for this recipe, as their mild flavors complement the vegetables and sauce.

Serve the fish and vegetable mixture over cooked rice or a bed of mashed potatoes to create a satisfying meal.

15. Blueberry Pancakes

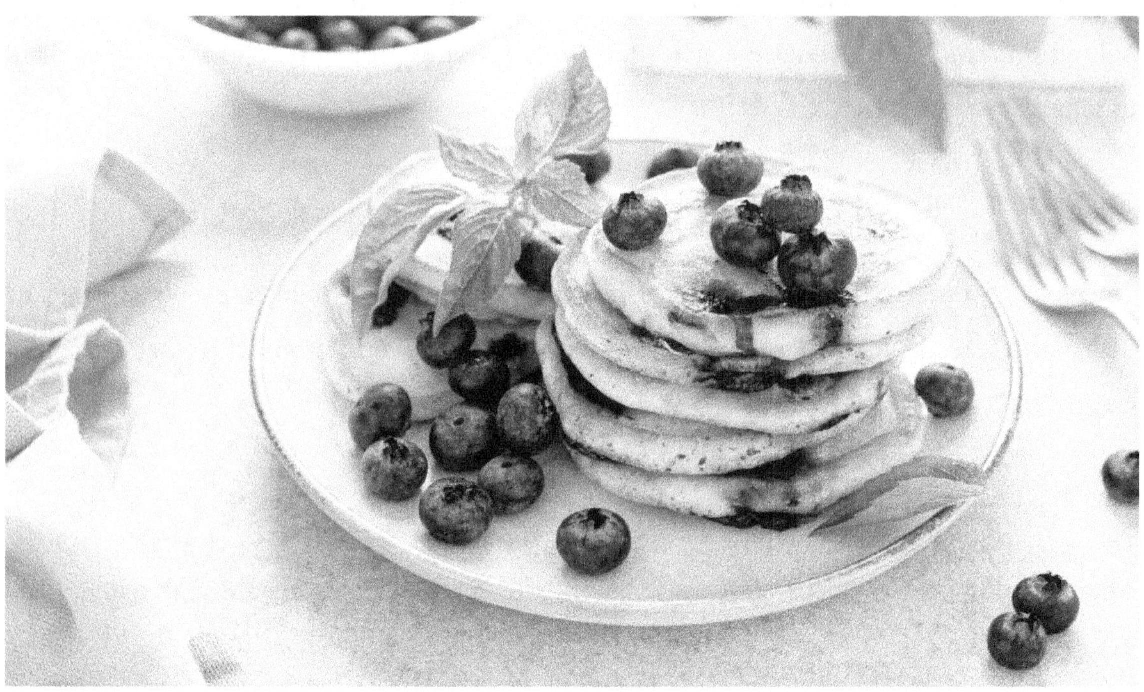

Blueberries are not just a fruit. They can be made into a fine and delicious pancake. If you like pancakes, now you can make them blueberry style.

Serve: 3

Prep Time: 30 minutes

List of Ingredients:

- 1/2 cup of arrowroot powder
- 1 pinch of sea salt
- 1/2 teaspoon of baking soda
- 1/2 teaspoon of yeast
- 1/2 cup of coconut flour
- 1/2 tablespoon of lemon juice
- 1-pint of blueberries
- 1 teaspoon of vanilla extract
- 3 omega-3 fresh eggs
- 1 teaspoon of cinnamon
- 1/4 cup of coconut oil
- 1/4 cup of walnuts, roughly chopped
- 1 teaspoon of vanilla extract

sssssssssssssssssss

Methods:

Step 1: Whisking the Wet Ingredients

In a mixing bowl, whisk the eggs until well-beaten. Add in the vanilla extract, lemon juice, and almond milk. Ensure thorough mixing to create a cohesive wet mixture.

Step 2: Blending the Dry Ingredients

In another bowl, combine the arrowroot, salt, yeast, baking powder, cinnamon, and coconut flour. This dry mixture forms the foundation for your pancake batter.

Step 3: Combining Wet and Dry Mixtures

Gradually incorporate the wet mixture into the dry mixture while continuously whisking. This step ensures even distribution of the ingredients and prevents lumps from forming in the batter.

Step 4: Adding Chopped Walnuts

Gently fold in the chopped walnuts to the pancake batter. This addition contributes a satisfying crunch and nutty flavor to the pancakes.

Step 5: Cooking the Pancakes

Heat a saucepan over medium heat and grease it with coconut oil. Once the oil is hot, ladle portions of the pancake batter onto the pan. Cook the pancakes until bubbles form on the surface.

Step 6: Creating Blueberry Sauce

In a separate saucepan, simmer the fresh blueberries along with a small amount of water. This simple blueberry sauce complements the pancakes perfectly and adds a burst of fruity goodness.

Step 7: Serving the Pancakes

Once the blueberry sauce is ready and the pancakes are cooked, assemble your stack of pancakes. Pour the warm blueberry sauce generously over the stack, allowing it to cascade down the sides.

Fun Facts:

Blueberry pancakes are a delightful breakfast option that combines the wholesome goodness of pancakes with the burst of flavor from fresh blueberries.

Almond milk and coconut flour contribute to the pancakes' unique texture and flavor profile, making them suitable for those with dietary preferences or restrictions.

Did you know? Blueberries are rich in antioxidants and are often referred to as a "superfood" due to their potential health benefits.

Suggestions:

Top your stack of blueberry pancakes with a dollop of Greek yogurt, a drizzle of honey, or a sprinkle of chopped nuts for added texture and flavor.

Serve these pancakes alongside a side of crispy bacon or scrambled eggs to create a balanced and satisfying breakfast spread.

16. Crispy Papillote of Whiting

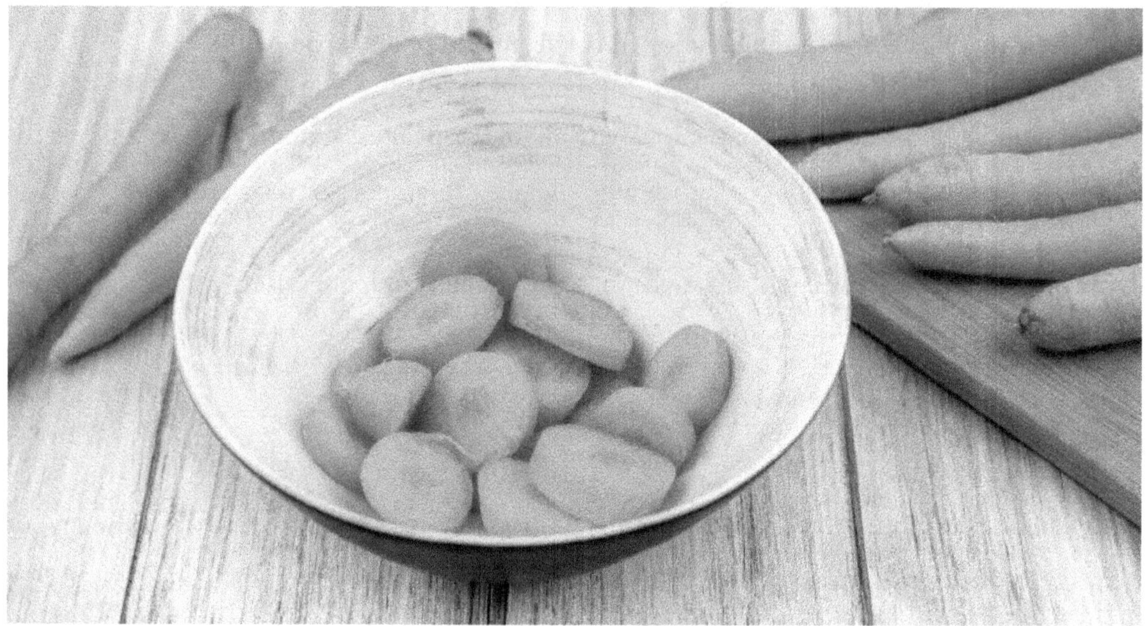

Instead of using the traditional cooking paper for the papillote, use some filo pastry; a very interesting change. Cooking in papillote is always very easy and most of the results are very good. Serve it with a nice salad and some quarters of lemon for garnish.

Serve: 4

Prep Time: 25 minutes

List of Ingredients:

- 1 leek, finely sliced
- 5 garlic cloves, thinly chopped
- Salt and pepper
- 4 whiting filets
- 3 carrots, finely slice
- 4 sheets of filo pastry
- 4 tablespoons of white wine
- 1 sprig of thyme

sssssssssssssssssss

Methods:

Step 1: Preheating the Oven

Begin by preheating the oven to 350°F (175°C). This temperature will ensure that the papillotes cook evenly and develop a crispy texture.

Step 2: Seasoning the Fish

Season both sides of the fish filets with your preferred seasonings. Seasoning with salt, pepper, and herbs of your choice will enhance the flavor of the whiting filets.

Step 3: Preparing the Filo Pastry Sheets

Lay out the filo pastry sheets on a clean work surface. Filo pastry is delicate, so handle it gently to prevent tearing.

Step 4: Assembling the Papillotes

Place a whiting filet on each filo pastry sheet. This will be the centerpiece of the papillotes.

Distribute the leeks, carrots, and garlic evenly around the fish filets. These vegetables will add flavor and complement the fish.

Step 5: Adding Flavor Elements

Pour a splash of white wine over each fish filet. This will infuse the fish with a delicate flavor as it bakes.

Sprinkle fresh thyme leaves over the fish. Thyme's aromatic qualities will enhance the overall taste of the dish.

Step 6: Folding and Securing

Gently fold the edges of the filo pastry over the fish and vegetables, creating a neat packet. Secure the ends of the papillotes by tying them with kitchen string or securing them with wooden picks.

Step 7: Brushing with Olive Oil

Brush the exterior of the papillotes with olive oil. This step adds a touch of richness and helps the pastry develop a crispy texture during baking.

Step 8: Baking the Papillotes

Place the prepared papillotes on a baking sheet and place them in the preheated oven. Allow them to bake for about 10 minutes, ensuring that the filo pastry becomes golden and crispy.

Step 9: Serving the Dish

Once the papillotes are cooked and the filo pastry is crispy, carefully remove them from the oven.

Serve the crispy papillotes of whiting hot, unwrapping the delicate packages to reveal the aromatic and flavorful fish and vegetables inside.

Fun Facts:

Papillote is a French cooking technique that involves wrapping food in parchment paper or other suitable materials and baking it. This method helps to retain flavors and moisture while cooking.

Whiting is a delicate and mild-flavored fish that cooks quickly and pairs well with various seasonings and vegetables.

Did you know? The term "papillote" comes from the French word for "butterfly," referring to the folded shape of the parchment paper resembling butterfly wings.

Suggestions:

Enhance the flavors by adding fresh herbs like rosemary or dill to the papillotes before baking.

For an added burst of citrusy flavor, include thin slices of lemon or lime alongside the fish and vegetables.

Serve the papillotes with a side of steamed rice, quinoa, or a mixed green salad to create a balanced and satisfying meal.

17. Avocado Caesar Salad

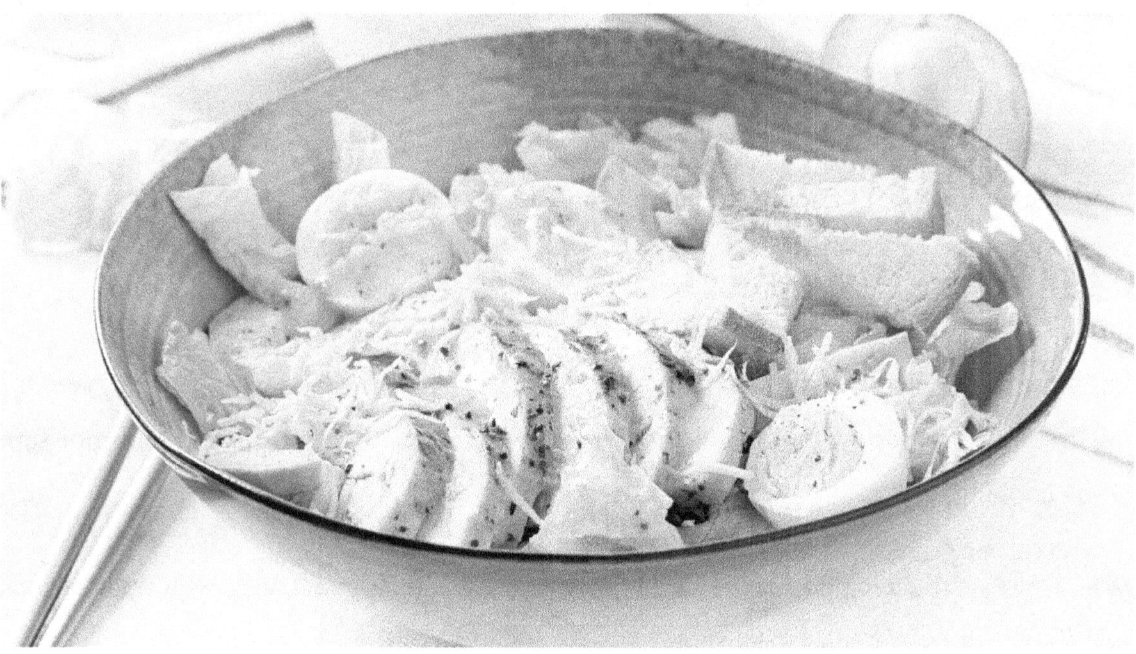

This is a different way of doing the classic Caesar salad recipe. Remember, instead of avocado, you can always add some grilled chicken too or even both. You can do the croutons a day before if you have time barriers, but for myself, I prefer doing them on the same day - they are crustier and not hard.

Serve: 4

Prep Time: 30 minutes

List of Ingredients:

- 2 tablespoons of parsley, finely chopped
- 4 slices of bread, cut into cubes
- 2 egg yolks
- 8 tablespoons of olive oil
- 1 tablespoon of mustard
- 8 anchovies
- 4 tablespoons of parmesan, grated
- Salt and pepper
- 1 romaine lettuce
- 2 avocados, sliced
- 1 red onion, sliced
- 3 garlic cloves, thinly chopped

sssssssssssssssssss

Methods:

Step 1: Preparing the Croutons

Warm up two tablespoons of olive oil in a frying pan over medium heat.

Add two garlic cloves and the parsley, and cook for 2 to 3 minutes to infuse the oil with flavor.

Add the small bread cubes and cook until they turn golden brown. Set the croutons aside.

Step 2: Making the Dressing

In a blender, combine the rest of the garlic, anchovies, and mustard.

Add the egg yolks and start blending. Gradually pour in the remaining olive oil until the mixture becomes smooth and creamy. Season the dressing to taste, and adjust the consistency by adding more olive oil if desired.

Step 3: Assembling the Salad

In a large bowl, mix the romaine lettuce with the prepared dressing, ensuring even coating.

Add the red onion and the previously made croutons to the lettuce, adding crunch and flavor to the salad.

Step 4: Incorporating Avocado

Gently fold in the avocado pieces, being careful not to mash them. Avocado adds a creamy texture and a boost of nutrition to the salad.

Step 5: Final Touch and Serving

Sprinkle the salad with grated Parmesan cheese for a savory kick and added richness.

Serve the Avocado Caesar Salad as a delicious side or main dish, enjoyed by itself or paired with grilled protein of your choice.

Fun Facts:

Caesar salad is a classic and beloved dish that originated in Tijuana, Mexico, by chef Caesar Cardini in the 1920s.

The creamy dressing typically includes ingredients like garlic, anchovies, and Parmesan cheese, providing a rich and flavorful experience.

Avocado is a nutritious addition, contributing healthy fats, vitamins, and a creamy texture to the salad.

Suggestions:

For a protein boost, consider adding grilled chicken, shrimp, or tofu to turn this side dish into a satisfying main course.

Experiment with different types of lettuce, such as kale or spinach, for a unique twist on the traditional romaine base.

Customize the salad by incorporating additional toppings like cherry tomatoes, crumbled bacon, or roasted nuts.

18. Roasted Veggies

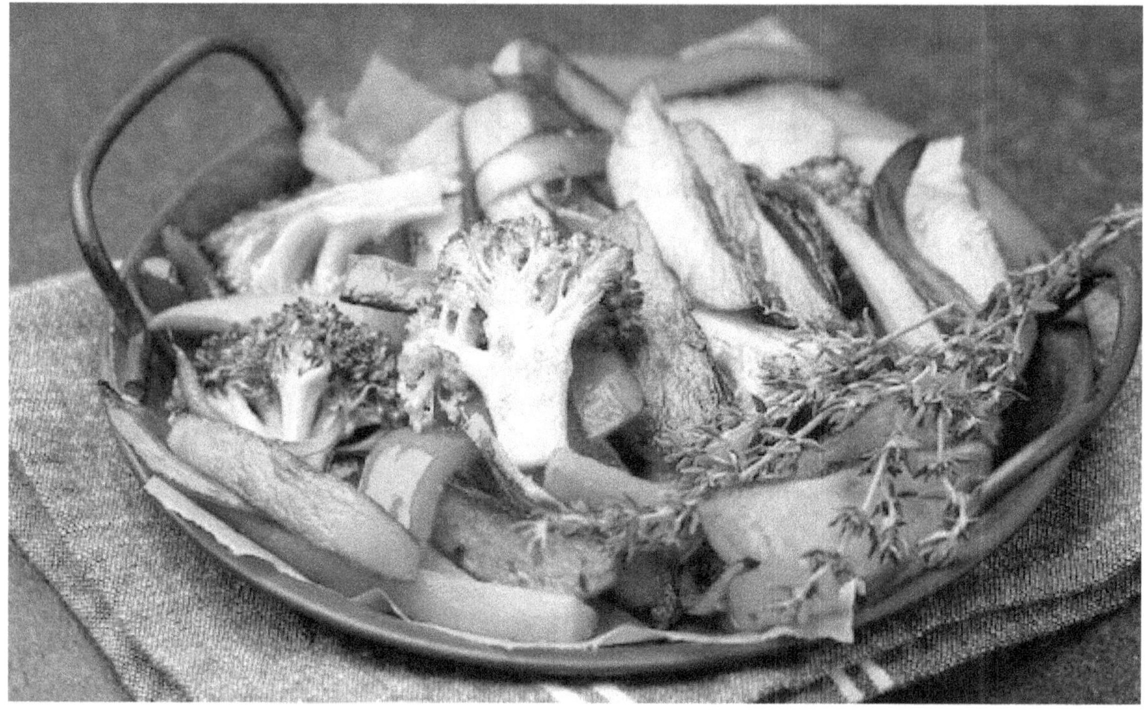

Roasted vegetables are a great way to get some of the goodness of your vegetables without having to cook them on the stove because they are easy to throw in the oven and when they come out, they taste like you spent hours preparing them.

Serve: 2

Prep Time: 50 minutes

List of Ingredients:

- 1 tablespoon of extra-virgin olive oil
- 6 cloves of garlic
- 3/4 teaspoon of kosher salt
- 2 tablespoons of fresh rosemary needles
- 1/2 lb. of turnips
- 1/2 lb. of carrots
- 1/2 lb. of parsnips
- 2 shallots, peeled
- 1/4 teaspoon of ground black pepper

sssssssssssssssssss

Methods:

Step 1: Preparing the Veggies

Begin by cutting the turnips, carrots, parsnips, and shallots into bite-sized pieces. This ensures even cooking and easy serving.

Step 2: Roasting the Veggies

Preheat the oven to 400°F (200°C), creating the ideal temperature for roasting vegetables.

In a baking dish, mix the cut vegetables with extra-virgin olive oil, minced garlic, kosher salt, and fresh rosemary needles. This combination infuses the veggies with rich flavors and aromas.

Place the baking dish in the preheated oven and roast the vegetables for about 25 minutes, or until they turn brown and become tender.

Step 3: Roasting and Serving

After the initial 25 minutes, take the baking dish out of the oven and give the veggies a toss. This ensures even roasting and browning.

Return the baking dish to the oven and continue roasting for an additional 20 to 25 minutes. This final step brings out the veggies' natural sweetness and adds a delightful caramelized crust.

Once the roasted veggies are golden brown and tender, remove them from the oven.

Fun Facts:

Roasting vegetables enhances their natural flavors and creates a delicious caramelized exterior.

Fresh rosemary needles not only add flavor but also release a wonderful aroma when roasted.

This dish is versatile and can be customized with your favorite vegetables and herbs.

Suggestions:

Add a sprinkle of grated Parmesan cheese over the roasted veggies before serving for an extra burst of flavor.

Drizzle a balsamic reduction or lemon juice over the roasted vegetables for a tangy twist.

Serve these roasted veggies as a side dish alongside grilled chicken or baked fish for a complete meal.

19. My 'Ota'ika

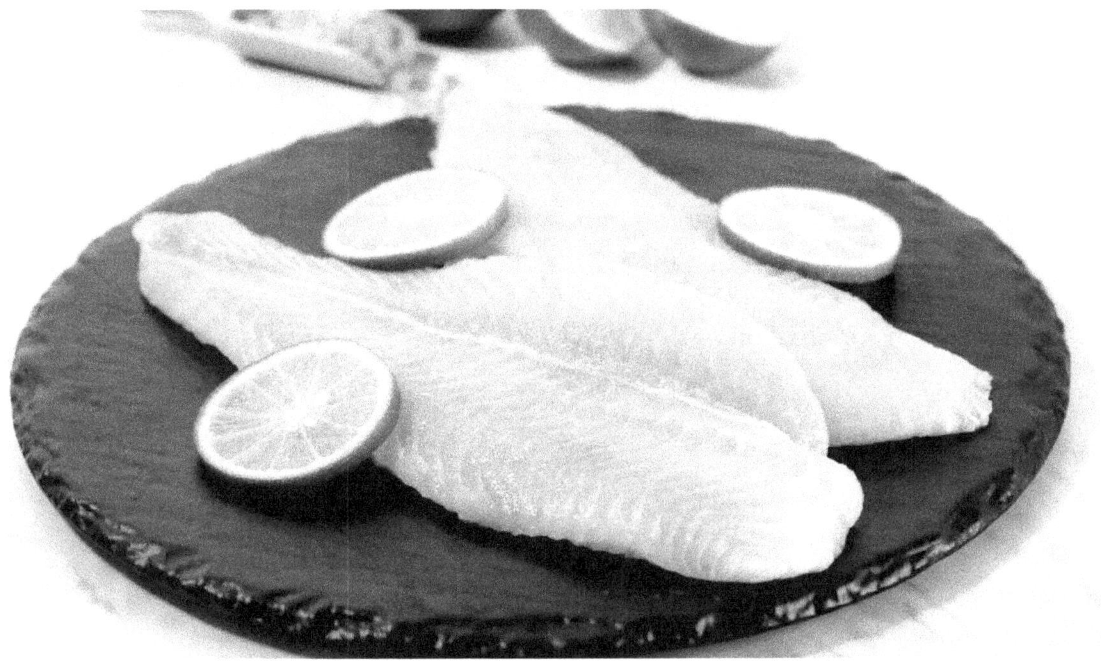

The fish is raw so try to choose a variety of fish that has a firm flesh, such as tuna, sea bream, etc. If you place the fish in the freezer for a few minutes before cutting, you will find the process to be very easy. Serve with a green salad on the side. This recipe originated from Tahiti.

Serve: 6

Prep Time: 25 minutes

List of Ingredients:

- ½ a cucumber
- 1 onion
- 6 tablespoons of coconut, grated
- Salt and pepper
- 5 lb. of fresh fish
- 6 limes, juiced
- 3 tablespoons of olive oil
- 2 tomatoes
- 2 carrots

sssssssssssssssssss

Methods:

Step 1: Preparing the Fish

Begin by cutting the fish into thin strips and placing them in a large bowl.

Step 2: Marinating the Fish

Fill the bowl with salty water and refrigerate it. This process helps to firm up the fish and enhances its flavor.

Step 3: Preparing the Vegetables

Peel and finely dice the onion, and do the same with the tomatoes.

Cut the cucumber into small dice and grate the carrots. Keep them aside.

Grate the coconut and set it aside as well.

Step 4: Assembling the Dish

Drain and rinse the fish with clear water to remove excess salt.

Squeeze the lime juice onto the fish and add the olive oil. Mix well to ensure even distribution of flavors and seasonings.

Step 5: Adding Fresh Ingredients

Incorporate the diced cucumber, tomatoes, onion, and grated carrots to the fish mixture.

Step 6: Adding Coconut Flavor

Add the grated coconut to the mixture and gently combine all the ingredients.

Step 7: Final Touch and Chilling

Season the dish according to your taste preferences.

Allow the flavors to meld by placing the fish mixture in the refrigerator before serving.

Fun Facts:

'Ota'ika is a traditional dish known for its fresh and vibrant flavors.

This dish hails from the Polynesian islands and often features fresh seafood and tropical ingredients.

'Ota'ika is a wonderful representation of the culinary culture of the Pacific Islands.

Suggestions:

Enjoy 'Ota'ika as a refreshing appetizer or light meal on a warm day.

Customize the dish by adding your favorite tropical fruits or herbs for a unique twist.

Serve 'Ota'ika with toasted bread or tortilla chips for added texture and crunch.

20. Asian Zucchini Salad

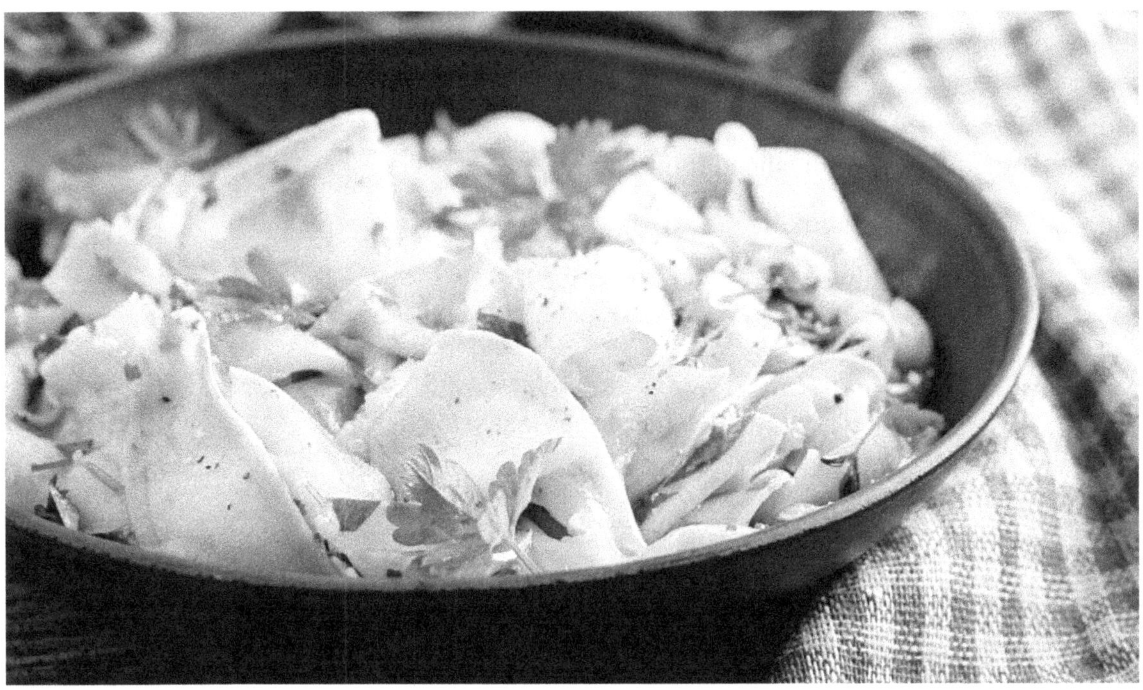

There are many ways you can prepare zucchini to make it into a salad. This recipe is one of the most popular. It is full of veggies and all kinds of different spices that will help it taste better than just all about zucchini.

Serve: 4

Prep Time: 2 hours 20 minutes

List of Ingredients:

- 1/3 cup of rice vinegar
- 1 teaspoon of Stevia drops
- 1 cup of almonds, sliced
- 1 medium zucchini, sliced thinly into spirals
- 3/4 cup of avocado oil
- 1 cup of sunflower seeds, shells removed
- 1 lb. of cabbage, shredded

sssssssssssssssssss

Methods:

Step 1: Preparing Zucchini Spirals

Begin by cutting the zucchini spirals into smaller, manageable pieces. Set the zucchini aside for later use.

Step 2: Combining Salad Ingredients

In a large bowl, combine the almonds, sunflower seeds, and cabbage from the List of Ingredients. Make sure to mix these ingredients well to distribute flavors and textures evenly.

Step 3: Adding Zucchini

Add the prepared zucchini spirals to the bowl containing the almond, sunflower seed, and cabbage mixture. The zucchini will add a refreshing crunch to the salad.

Step 4: Making the Dressing

In a separate small bowl, whisk together the vinegar, stevia, and oil until well combined. This dressing will contribute a balanced blend of tanginess and sweetness to the salad.

Step 5: Dressing the Salad

Drizzle the prepared vinegar mixture over the zucchini and cabbage mixture in the large bowl. Toss the salad thoroughly to ensure that all the ingredients are coated with the dressing.

Step 6: Chilling the Salad

Once the salad is dressed, refrigerate it for about 2 hours before serving. Chilling the salad allows the flavors to meld together and enhances its overall taste.

Fun Facts:

Asian Zucchini Salad offers a refreshing and light dish that combines crunchy vegetables, zesty dressing, and a delightful blend of textures and flavors.

This salad incorporates zucchini spirals, almonds, sunflower seeds, and cabbage for a nutrient-rich and satisfying meal.

The Asian-inspired dressing, featuring vinegar and stevia, adds a tangy and slightly sweet element to the dish.

Suggestions:

Enhance the salad's protein content by adding grilled tofu, edamame, or cooked chicken slices.

Customize the salad by including other colorful vegetables such as bell peppers, shredded carrots, or sliced radishes for added visual appeal.

Garnish the salad with fresh chopped cilantro, mint leaves, or sesame seeds to enhance its taste and presentation.

21. Savory Chicken and Lentil Soup

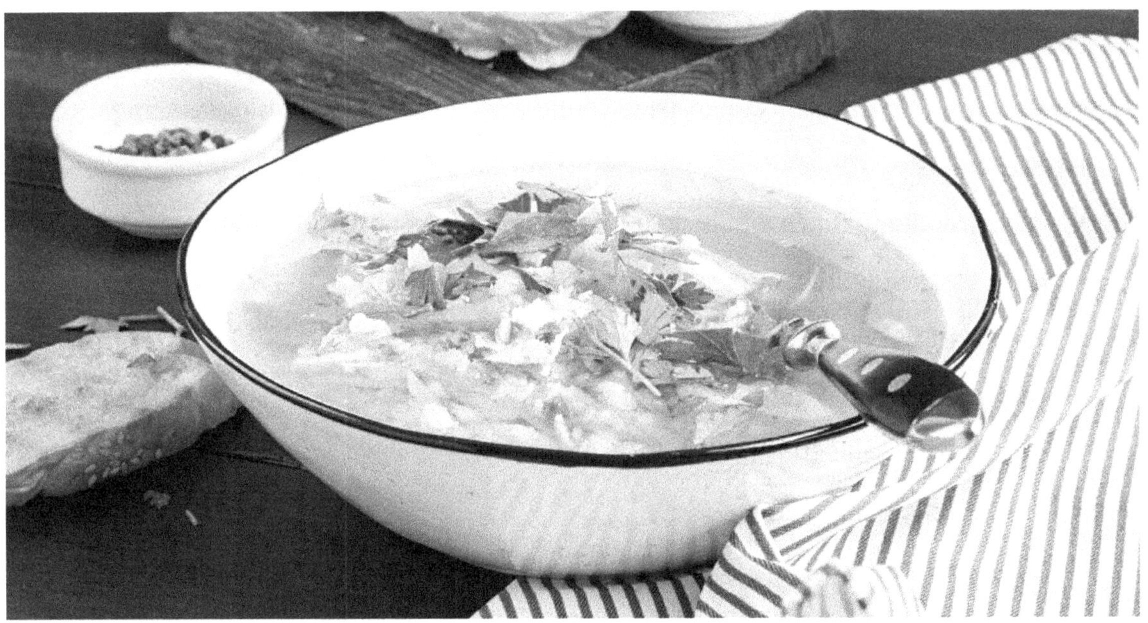

Lentils are another great source of protein. You can mix them up with some chicken and make them into a delicious soup.

Serve: 4

Prep Time: 1 hour

List of Ingredients:

- 1/4 cup of cilantro, chopped or minced
- 1 tablespoon of chicken stock
- 1/4 teaspoon of Spanish paprika, ground annatto seed, or Sazon seasoning
- salt, to taste
- 12 oz. or about 3 pcs. of chicken thighs, remove bones, skin, and fat
- 1 lb. of dried lentils
- 8 cups of water
- 3 cloves of garlic, minced
- 2 scallions, minced
- 1 ripe tomato, minced
- 1 onion, minced
- 1 teaspoon of cumin
- 1 teaspoon of garlic powder
- 1/4 teaspoon of oregano

ssssssssssssssssssss

Methods:

Step 1: Preparing the Base

In a large pot, combine dried lentils, chicken thighs (bones, skin, and fat removed), water, and chicken stock. This flavorful base sets the stage for a hearty and nourishing soup.

Step 2: Simmering and Cooking

Cover the pot and bring the mixture to a boil over medium-low heat. Let it simmer for approximately 20 minutes or until the chicken thighs are fully cooked and tender.

Step 3: Shredding Chicken

Carefully remove the cooked chicken thighs from the pot and use two forks to shred the meat. Return the shredded chicken to the pot. This step adds a delightful texture and additional protein to the soup.

Step 4: Flavorful Enhancements

Add minced garlic, scallions, ripe tomato, onion, cumin, garlic powder, and oregano to the pot. These ingredients contribute layers of flavor that elevate the overall taste of the soup.

Step 5: Cooking Lentils

Allow the soup to continue simmering for about 25 minutes or until the lentils are tender and fully cooked. If the soup thickens too much, you can adjust the consistency by adding more water.

Step 6: Seasoning and Serving

Taste the soup and season with salt according to your preference. Salt enhances the flavors and balances the dish.

Ladle the savory chicken and lentil soup into bowls and garnish with chopped cilantro. Serve the soup while it's hot and enjoy a comforting and satisfying meal.

Fun Facts:

Lentils are a fantastic source of plant-based protein and dietary fiber, making this soup both nutritious and satisfying.

The combination of aromatic spices like cumin, garlic powder, and oregano adds depth and flavor to the soup, creating a delightful and comforting meal.

Suggestions:

Customize the soup by adding your favorite vegetables like carrots, celery, or spinach for extra nutrients and color.

Serve the soup with a squeeze of fresh lemon juice for a tangy kick and a burst of brightness.

Enjoy this soup with a side of crusty bread or a simple green salad for a well-rounded meal.

22. Pork Filet with Leeks and Caramelized Apple

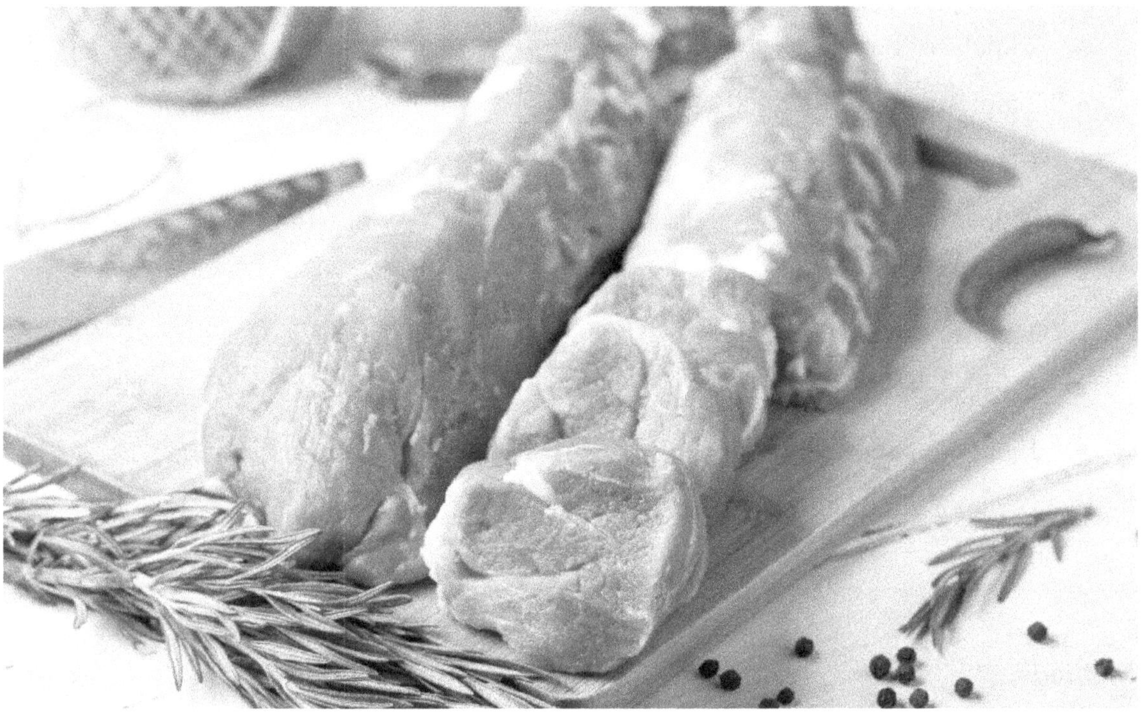

The leek is one of a few vegetables that can be found all year round thanks to its different varieties and also because it is resistant to cold winters. It is in this season when the leek is the most useful because it is very rich in vitamins and minerals.

Serve: 4

Prep Time: 40 minutes

List of Ingredients:

- 4 tablespoons of red wine
- 2 knobs of butter
- 2 tablespoons of olive oil
- 1 tablespoon of honey
- Pepper and salt
- 4 pork filets or tenderloins
- 4 apples, cut in quarters
- 2 leeks, shredded
- 1 garlic clove, finely chopped
- ¾ cup of chicken stock

ssssssssssssssssssss

Methods:

Step 1: Caramelizing the Apples

Warm up the butter in a large frying pan over medium heat. This step helps create a smooth base for caramelizing the apples.

Add honey to the pan and mix well. Then, introduce the apple slices into the mixture. The honey will add sweetness to the apples as they caramelize.

Cook the apples gently over low heat, frequently turning them to ensure even caramelization. This process will take a few minutes, during which the apples will turn golden brown and fragrant.

Once the apples are beautifully caramelized, remove them from the heat and set them aside to cool down. The caramelized apples will provide a sweet and slightly tangy contrast to the savory pork and leeks.

Step 2: Cooking the Pork Fillet

Heat olive oil in another frying pan over medium heat. The olive oil will help prevent the pork filet from sticking to the pan and ensure even cooking.

Add minced garlic to the pan and cook for about 2 minutes, releasing its aromatic flavor into the oil.

Place the pork filet into the pan and cook thoroughly on both sides until it reaches your desired level of doneness. The pork will turn tender and juicy as it cooks.

Once the pork filet is cooked, remove it from the pan and keep it warm by covering it with foil or placing it in a slightly warmed oven.

Step 3: Creating the Leek Sauce

Deglaze the pan with red wine, using a spatula to scrape up any flavorful bits from the bottom. This process adds depth to the sauce by incorporating the rich flavors from the pan.

Pour in the chicken stock and bring the mixture to a simmer over medium heat. The chicken stock will form the base of the sauce and contribute savory notes to the dish.

Add the sliced leeks to the pan and cook until the liquid reduces and thickens slightly, creating a luscious sauce with a balanced consistency.

Step 4: Plating and Serving

To assemble the dish, start by placing a bed of cooked leeks on each plate. The leeks will provide a flavorful base for the pork and apples.

Arrange the cooked pork filet on top of the leeks, showcasing its tender texture and savory flavor.

Spoon the caramelized apples over the pork, adding a touch of sweetness and a burst of fruity taste.

Enjoy this harmonious combination of flavors and textures as you savor each bite of Pork Fillet with Leeks and Caramelized Apple.

Fun Facts:

This dish combines the savory flavors of pork filet and leeks with the sweetness of caramelized apples, creating a delightful balance of taste.

Caramelizing apples with honey adds a touch of natural sweetness and enhances their flavor.

Suggestions:

Serve this elegant dish with a side of creamy mashed potatoes or steamed rice to complement the flavors.

For added texture, consider sprinkling toasted nuts, such as chopped walnuts or pecans, over the dish before serving.

To enhance the presentation, garnish the plate with a sprinkle of chopped fresh herbs, such as parsley or chives.

23. Fresh Asparagus Salad

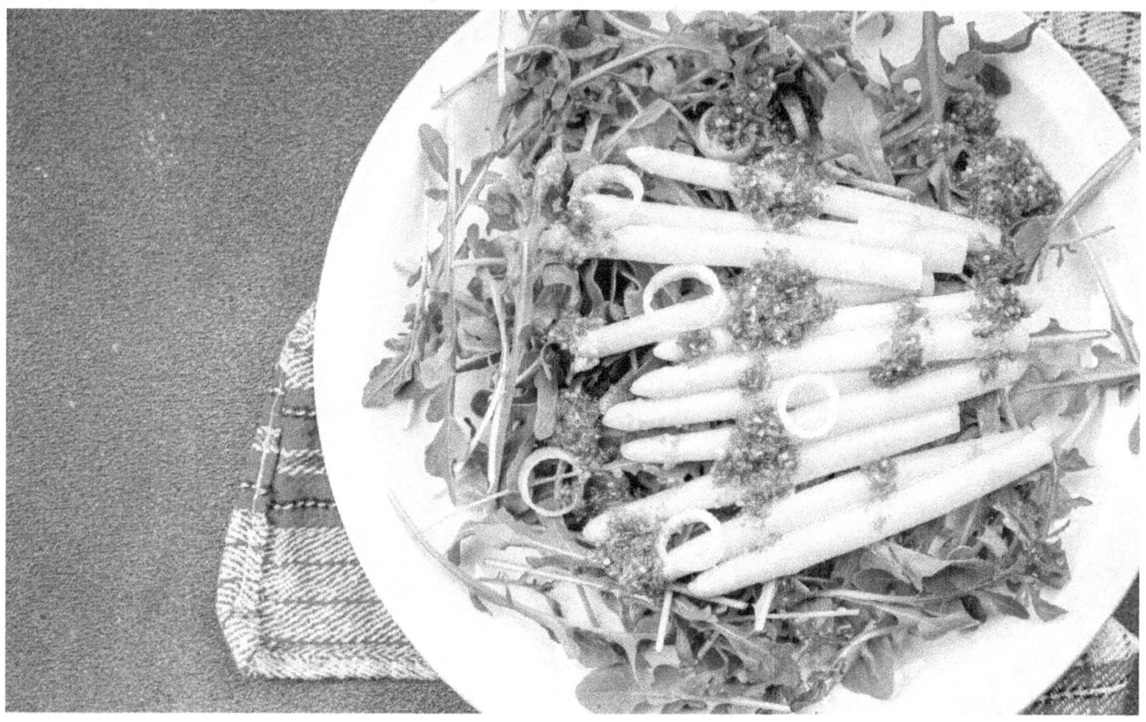

Asparagus has a very mild taste and has been known to be eaten by those that are not fond of much seasoning. A fresh asparagus salad can be made with whatever vegetables you prefer, but no matter what you do the asparagus will just complement the flavor of whatever else you use them with.

Serve: 4

Prep Time: 1 hour 10 minutes

List of Ingredients:

- 4 teaspoons of lemon juice
- 2 tablespoons of sea salt
- Virgin olive oil
- 2 lbs. of asparagus
- 1/3 cup of hazelnuts
- 4 cups of arugula
- 1 teaspoon of ground pepper

sssssssssssssssssss

Methods:

Step 1: Preparing Hazelnuts

Preheat your oven to 400°F (200°C).

Place the hazelnuts on a baking tray lined with parchment paper and roast them in the oven for about 7 minutes. Roasting the hazelnuts brings out their rich flavor and adds a satisfying crunch.

Step 2: Peeling and Chopping Hazelnuts (Optional)

Once roasted, transfer the hazelnuts to a plate. If desired, you can remove the skins for a smoother texture by wrapping the nuts in a towel and rubbing them vigorously.

Coarsely chop the hazelnuts after peeling, ensuring they're ready to be added to the salad.

Step 3: Roasting Asparagus

Trim the tough ends of the asparagus stalks to prepare them for roasting.

Place the trimmed asparagus on the same baking sheet used for the hazelnuts. Drizzle 1 tablespoon of olive oil and sprinkle 1/2 teaspoon of salt over the asparagus.

Roast the asparagus in the preheated oven for approximately 8 minutes, allowing them to become tender and slightly crispy.

Step 4: Creating Dressing

In a mixing bowl, whisk together ground pepper, salt, remaining olive oil, and fresh lemon juice. This dressing adds a zesty and tangy element to the salad.

Step 5: Assembling the Salad

Place the arugula in a medium bowl and drizzle about half of the prepared dressing over the greens. Toss the arugula until it's evenly coated with the dressing.

Transfer the dressed arugula onto a serving platter, creating the base of the salad.

Step 6: Arranging Asparagus and Hazelnuts

Arrange the roasted asparagus stalks on top of the arugula bed, creating an appealing presentation.

Sprinkle the peeled and chopped hazelnuts over the salad, adding a delightful nutty crunch.

Fun Facts:

Asparagus is a nutrient-rich vegetable packed with vitamins and minerals, making it a healthy addition to your salad.

Roasting hazelnuts enhances their flavor and adds a delightful crunch to the salad.

Suggestions:

For an extra burst of flavor, consider adding crumbled feta or goat cheese to the salad.

To add a touch of sweetness and contrast, toss in some dried cranberries or sliced strawberries.

This salad pairs well with grilled chicken, salmon, or tofu for a more substantial meal.

24. Mediterranean Peppers Salad

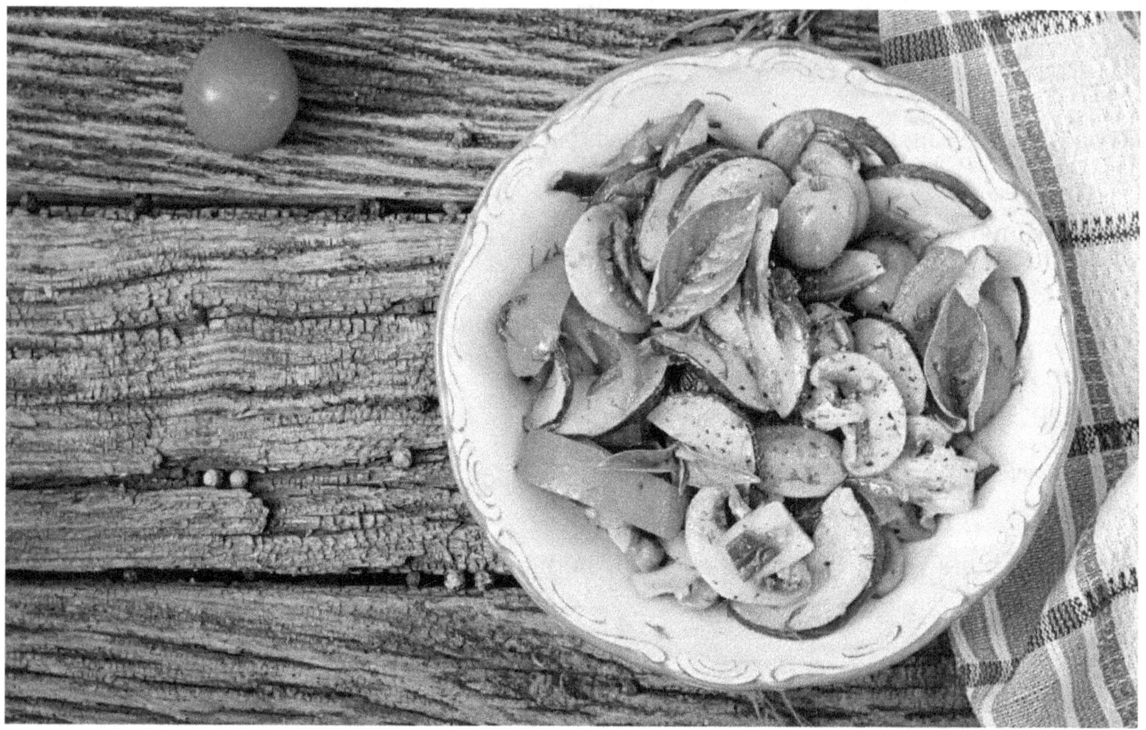

A full flavor recipe with so many different colors - this salad really gives you the warmth of the Mediterranean coast. You can add some cubes of cheese or some pieces of fish too, like tuna or salmon - the choice is yours. Eat as much as you want; it is very healthy for you.

Serve: 4

Prep Time: 45 minutes

List of Ingredients:

- 1 onion, thinly chopped
- 2 red peppers
- 2 garlic cloves, chopped
- 1 oz. of stoned black olive, halves
- 3 tablespoons of olive oil
- 1 tablespoon of basil
- Salt and pepper
- 2 yellow peppers
- 1 zucchini, sliced
- 10 cherry tomatoes, cut in halves
- 2 green peppers
- 1 tablespoon of balsamic vinegar

sssssssssssssssssss

Methods:

Step 1: Warming Olive Oil

Begin by heating the olive oil in a large frying pan. This step helps infuse the oil with its rich flavor, a signature of Mediterranean cuisine.

Step 2: Sweating Onion and Garlic

Add the onion and garlic to the pan and cook them until they become tender. Sweating the onion and garlic releases their aromatic flavors and enhances the base of the salad.

Step 3: Adding Peppers and Zucchini

Incorporate the colorful trio of green, red, and yellow peppers along with the zucchini. These vegetables contribute vibrant hues and various textures to the salad.

Step 4: Cooking on Low Heat

Cook the mixture over low heat for about 20 minutes, stirring occasionally. The gentle cooking process allows the flavors to meld together while preserving the vegetables' freshness.

Step 5: Introducing Olives and Cherry Tomatoes

Enhance the salad with the addition of black olives and cherry tomatoes. These ingredients offer a burst of flavor and contribute to the Mediterranean essence of the dish.

Step 6: Adding Basil and Vinegar

Incorporate fresh basil and vinegar to further enhance the taste profile. The basil provides an aromatic and herbaceous note, while the vinegar adds a tangy element.

Step 7: Seasoning and Mixing

Season the salad to taste, ensuring the flavors are well-balanced. Mix all the ingredients well, allowing the flavors to marry and creating a harmonious combination.

Step 8: Final Cooking and Serving

Cook the salad for an additional 5 minutes, stirring occasionally. This step allows the flavors to meld even further.

Serve the Mediterranean Peppers Salad either as a stand-alone dish or as a delightful accompaniment to a mixed salad, showcasing the vibrant and enticing flavors of the Mediterranean region.

Fun Facts:

Mediterranean cuisine is renowned for its emphasis on fresh vegetables, olive oil, and vibrant flavors.

Peppers, olives, and tomatoes are staples in Mediterranean cooking, contributing to the distinct and delicious taste of this salad.

Suggestions:

Serve this salad as a refreshing and colorful appetizer at your next gathering.

Pair the Mediterranean Peppers Salad with grilled chicken, fish, or crusty bread for a complete and satisfying meal.

Sprinkle crumbled feta cheese over the salad for added creaminess and tangy flavor.

25. Apricot-Glazed Salmon

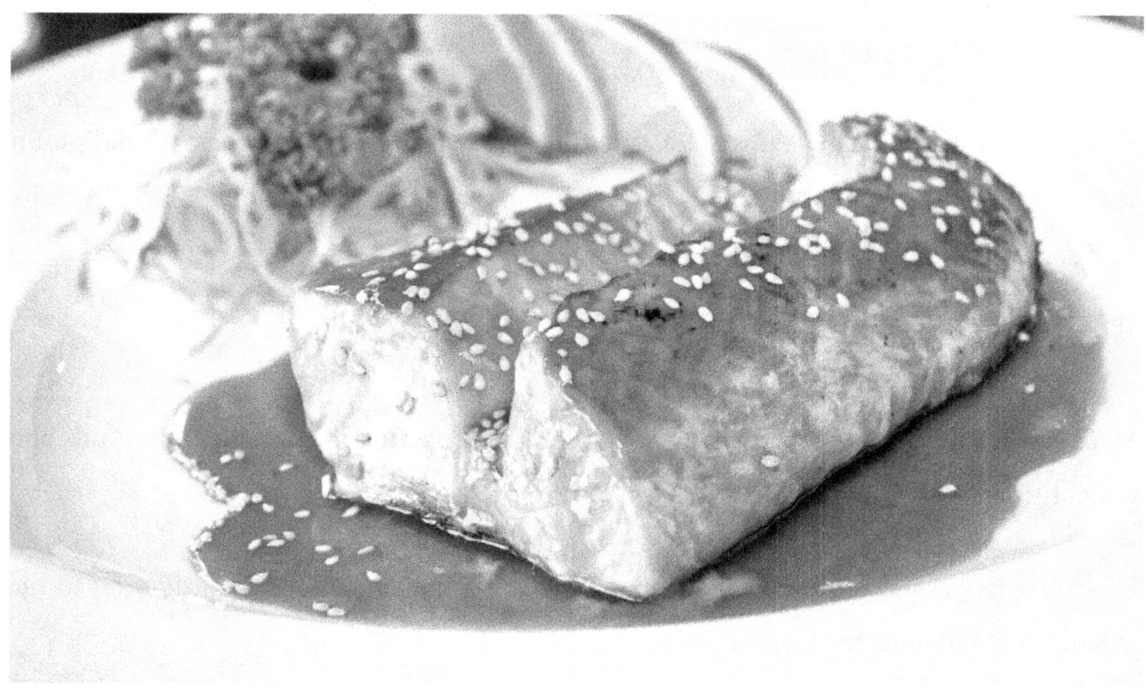

Salmon is a very popular fish for those that really like fish. A good thing about it is that it can be done in the oven, on the grill or in the frying pan. This recipe has a sweet apricot glaze that will give this salmon a whole new flavor.

Serve: 4

Prep Time: 1 hour 10 minutes

List of Ingredients:

- 1-1/3 pounds of wild salmon filets
- 1/2 cup of sodium-free vegetable broth
- 1 tablespoon of Dijon mustard
- 1/3 cup of 100% apricot fruit spread
- 1 teaspoon of minced garlic
- 1/4 teaspoon of crushed black pepper
- 1 tablespoon of virgin olive oil

sssssssssssssssssss

Methods:

Step 1: Preheating the Grill

Begin by preheating your grill over medium heat. Preheating ensures that the grill is ready to cook the salmon evenly and create those beautiful grill marks.

Step 2: Preparing Salmon

Pat the salmon dry using a paper towel to ensure a good sear. Cut the salmon into four slices, making it easier to grill and serve.

Step 3: Seasoning the Salmon

Sprinkle freshly ground black pepper on the skinless side of each salmon slice. This seasoning enhances the flavor of the fish and complements the sweetness of the apricot glaze.

Step 4: Wrapping with Aluminum Foil

Place each piece of seasoned salmon on a sheet of aluminum foil, skin side down. Wrap the foil around the salmon securely, ensuring that it's tightly sealed to prevent oil from leaking during grilling.

Step 5: Mixing the Apricot Glaze

In a bowl, combine the remaining ingredients to create the apricot glaze. This glaze will add a luscious layer of flavor and moisture to the grilled salmon.

Step 6: Applying the Glaze

Pour the apricot glaze mixture over the salmon slices, allowing the flavors to infuse while grilling.

Step 7: Grilling the Salmon

Place the foil-wrapped salmon on the preheated grill. Grill the salmon for approximately ten minutes, or until it reaches your desired level of doneness. The foil helps to steam the fish while trapping in the flavors.

Step 8: Cooling and Unwrapping

Once the salmon is cooked, carefully remove it from the grill and allow it to cool slightly before unwrapping the foil.

Step 9: Plating and Garnishing

Plate the grilled salmon slices nicely on serving dishes. Before serving, garnish with your favorite herbs, such as parsley, dill, or chives. These fresh herbs not only enhance the appearance but also contribute a delightful aroma and taste.

Fun Facts:

Salmon is a rich source of omega-3 fatty acids, which are beneficial for heart health and brain function.

Apricot glaze adds a delightful balance of sweetness and tanginess to the savory flavor of grilled salmon.

Suggestions:

Serve this apricot-glazed salmon with a side of steamed vegetables and quinoa for a well-rounded and nutritious meal.

Garnish the dish with chopped fresh herbs like parsley, dill, or chives to enhance the visual appeal and add a burst of fresh flavor.

For an extra layer of complexity, marinate the salmon in the apricot mixture for a few hours before grilling to allow the flavors to penetrate the fish.

26. Stuffed Zucchini with Beef and Grapes

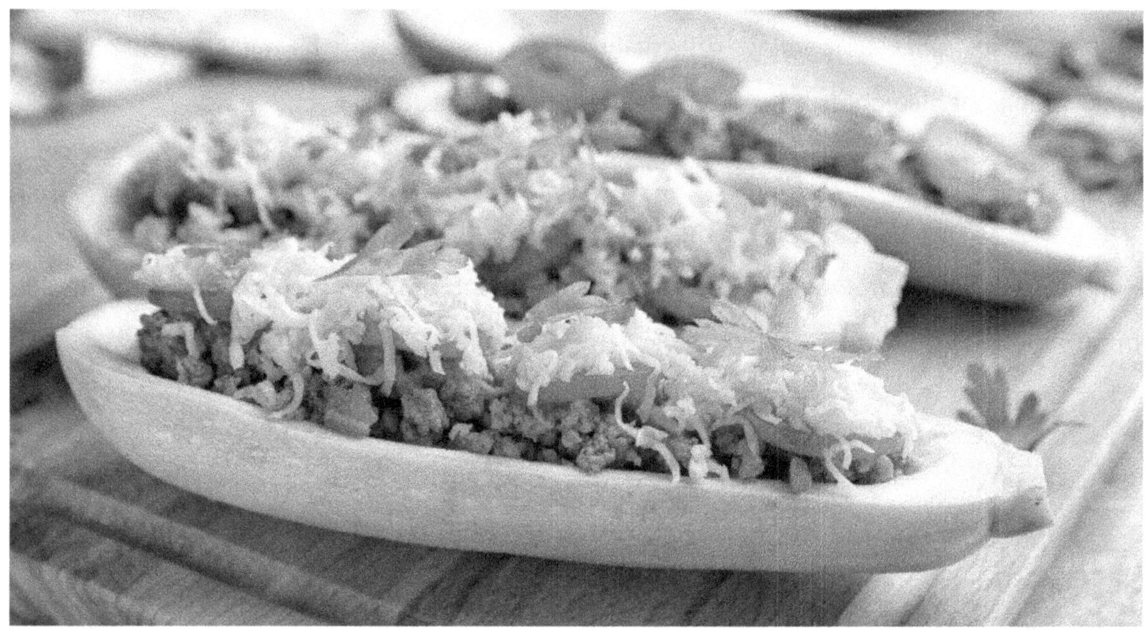

Meat is an essential part of our daily diet. Do not stop eating meat. Eat moderately and choose lean pieces, beef is a very nutritious food. It contains high-quality proteins; it is an excellent source of 12 vitamins and minerals as well, including iron and zinc.

Serve: 4

Prep Time: 1 hour 10 minutes

List of Ingredients:

- 2 garlic cloves, chopped
- 2 tomatoes, cut in pieces
- Salt and pepper
- 7/8 lb. of minced beef
- 8 round zucchini
- 1 onion, chopped
- 4 oz. of grapes, cut in halves
- 2 tablespoons of olive oil
- 7/8 cup of red wine
- 1 bunch of parsley, chopped

ssssssssssssssssss

Methods:

Step 1: Preheating the Oven

Begin by preheating the oven to 350°F (175°C). Preheating ensures that the oven is at the right temperature to cook the stuffed zucchini evenly.

Step 2: Cooking the Beef Mixture

Heat the olive oil in a frying pan over medium heat. Add the chopped onion and minced garlic, and sauté them until they become tender and aromatic.

Step 3: Adding and Cooking the Beef

Add the ground beef to the pan and cook for 3 to 4 minutes, breaking it into smaller pieces as it browns. The beef will contribute a hearty and savory element to the stuffing.

Step 4: Preparing the Zucchini

While the beef is cooking, prepare the zucchini by cutting off the tops and scooping out the insides, creating a hollow space to hold the stuffing.

Step 5: Enhancing the Filling

Incorporate the scooped-out zucchini, grapes, tomatoes, and red wine into the beef mixture. The grapes will add a delightful burst of sweetness, while the tomatoes and wine will enhance the overall flavor profile.

Step 6: Cooking the Filling

Allow the mixture to cook for an additional 5 minutes, allowing the flavors to meld together. Season the filling with your desired spices and herbs for added depth.

Step 7: Stuffing the Zucchini

Carefully stuff each hollowed zucchini with the flavorful beef and grape mixture. Place the zucchini tops back on as lids to keep the stuffing secure.

Step 8: Baking in the Oven

Arrange the stuffed zucchini in an oven-safe dish and place them in the preheated oven. Bake for 45 minutes, allowing the zucchini to soften and the flavors to infuse.

Step 9: Serving and Enjoying

Once the stuffed zucchini are tender and cooked through, remove them from the oven. Plate two stuffed zucchini per person, offering a satisfying and visually appealing portion.

Fun Facts:

Stuffed zucchini with beef and grapes is a unique and flavorful dish that combines the savory richness of beef with the natural sweetness of grapes.

This recipe transforms humble zucchini into an elegant and satisfying meal, making it a great choice for special occasions or family dinners.

Suggestions:

Garnish the stuffed zucchini with fresh herbs such as chopped parsley or basil for a burst of color and added flavor.

Consider using a mix of red and green grapes to add visual appeal to the dish and introduce a variety of flavors.

27. Smoked Trout and Apple Salad

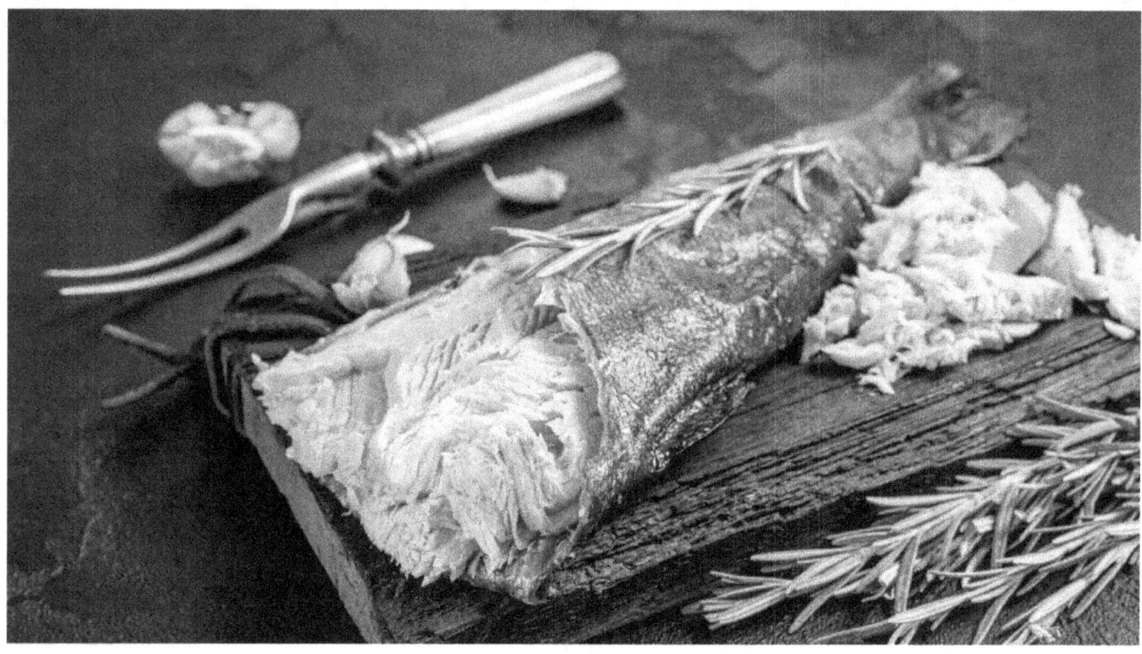

We never eat enough fruits during the day, so why not add them to our lunch or dinner. Here you have a perfect example of a salad and, to be honest, if you add some other fruit too, like pineapple, orange, grapefruit, they will all go perfectly with this salad. Enjoy!

Serve: 4

Prep Time: 20 minutes

List of Ingredients:

- 3 tablespoons of lemon juice
- 1 tablespoon of chives
- 2 tablespoons of Parmesan
- Salt and pepper
- 3 apples
- 6 oz. smoked trout
- ½ cup of natural yogurts
- 1 oak leaf salad or any other of your choice

sssssssssssssssssss

Methods:

Step 1: Preparing the Ingredients

Begin by cutting the apple into quarters and removing the cores. It's not necessary to peel the apples, as their skin adds texture and nutrition to the salad.

Step 2: Apple Preparation

Slice the apple quarters and place them in a bowl. To prevent browning, mix the sliced apples with two tablespoons of lemon juice. The lemon juice adds a tangy flavor and helps maintain the apple's color.

Step 3: Preparing the Oak Leaf Salad

Wash and drain the oak leaf salad, then break it into bite-sized pieces. Place the salad leaves in a large bowl, creating the base for your salad.

Step 4: Preparing the Trout

Carefully skin the smoked trout and check for any remaining bones. Gently flake the trout into large pieces and set them aside.

Step 5: Yogurt Dressing

In a small bowl, whisk together yogurt and one tablespoon of lemon juice. This tangy and creamy dressing will add a delightful contrast to the other ingredients.

Step 6: Assembling the Salad

Add the sliced apples and flaked trout to the oak leaf salad in the large bowl. This combination of sweet apples and smoky trout creates a well-balanced flavor profile.

Step 7: Dressing the Salad

Drizzle some of the yogurt dressing over the salad ingredients. Mix well to ensure even distribution of flavors and dressing.

Step 8: Serving

Plate the salad, and if desired, drizzle some extra yogurt dressing on top. The dressing not only adds creaminess but also complements the flavors of the trout and apples.

Fun Facts:

Smoked trout adds a delightful smoky flavor and a boost of protein to this refreshing salad.

Apples provide a sweet and crisp contrast to the savory trout and creamy yogurt dressing.

Suggestions:

Enhance the salad's flavors by adding toasted nuts, such as chopped walnuts or sliced almonds.

For added texture and color, toss in some dried cranberries or pomegranate seeds.

To add a delightful crunch to the salad, consider including toasted nuts or seeds of your choice.

Dried fruits like cranberries or pomegranate seeds can add pops of color and bursts of sweetness to the salad.

28. Spanish Style Fish Cutlets

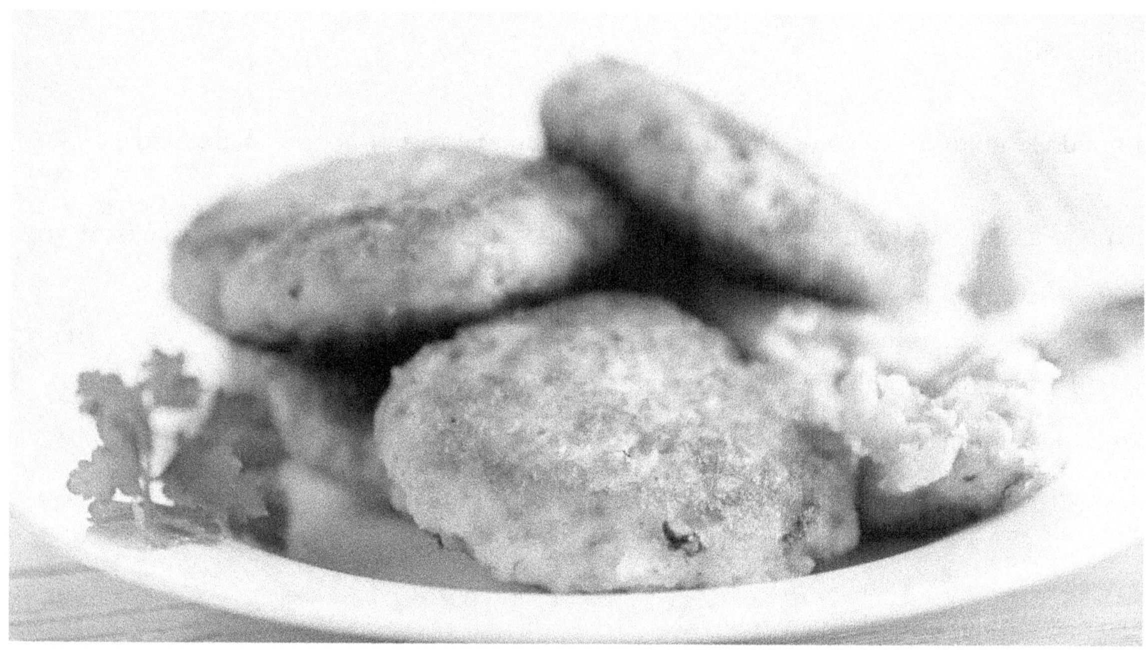

The mackerel is one of the fish so rich in omega 3. It also provides useful amounts of vitamins B and D, as well as several minerals. Like sardines, it is recommended to pregnant women. Available all year round and it is an easy fish to create a variety of recipes.

Serve: 4

Prep Time: 45 minutes

List of Ingredients:

- 1 oz. of almonds, slivered
- 1 tablespoon of green onions, chopped
- ½ teaspoon of paprika
- ½ teaspoon of lemon rind, grated
- 6 plum tomatoes
- Salt and pepper
- 4 jewfish cutlets
- 4 tablespoons of olive oil
- 1 tablespoon of parsley, chopped
- 3 garlic cloves, crushed

sssssssssssssssssss

Methods:

Step 1: Preheat the Oven

Preheat your oven to 350°F (175°C). The oven temperature is crucial to achieving the desired texture and flavor of the fish cutlets.

Step 2: Prepare the Fish

Brush both sides of the fish cutlets with olive oil. This step ensures the fish stays moist and doesn't stick to the oven tray during baking.

Step 3: Arrange the Cutlets

Place the prepared fish cutlets on an oven tray. Arranging them evenly on the tray allows for even cooking and browning.

Step 4: Prepare the Herb Mixture

In a bowl, combine the remaining olive oil with minced garlic. Mix in chopped parsley, paprika, sliced almonds, grated lemon rind, and chopped green onions. This flavorful mixture will be the topping for the fish cutlets.

Step 5: Top the Cutlets

Generously spoon the herb mixture over the top of each fish cutlet on the oven tray. The mixture adds a burst of aromatic flavors and enhances the presentation.

Step 6: Add Plum Tomatoes

Place plum tomatoes on the side of the fish cutlets on the oven tray. The roasted tomatoes will complement the fish and add a juicy element to the dish.

Step 7: Bake in the Oven

Place the oven tray with the fish cutlets and tomatoes in the preheated oven. Bake for approximately 20 minutes. Keep an eye on the fish to ensure it is cooked to your desired level of doneness.

Step 8: Check for Doneness

After 20 minutes, check the fish for doneness. The flesh should be opaque and easily flake with a fork. If needed, you can extend the cooking time slightly.

Fun Facts:

Spanish cuisine is known for its bold flavors and use of fresh ingredients, making this dish a delightful representation of the culinary culture.

Almonds and paprika are common ingredients in Spanish cooking, adding depth and complexity to the flavor profile of these fish cutlets.

Suggestions:

Serve the fish cutlets with a side of sautéed vegetables or a fresh salad for a well-balanced meal.

Experiment with different types of fish, such as cod, haddock, or snapper, to explore various flavor combinations.

29. Green Salad

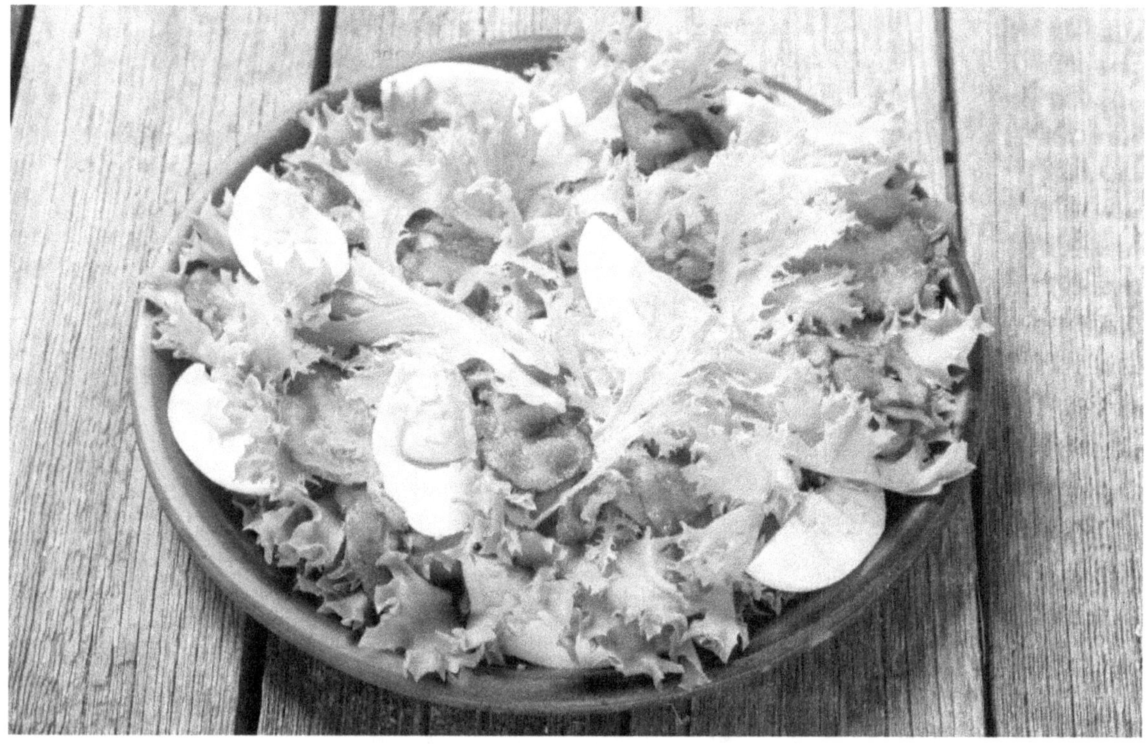

A green salad is supposed to be pretty basic. The ones in the restaurants have all kinds of fancy things added to them, such as bacon bits, sun dried tomatoes, pickles and other dressings that could make them a very unhealthy choice. This recipe will keep them healthy.

Serve: 3

Prep Time: 30 minutes

List of Ingredients:

- 2 tablespoons of shelled sunflower seeds
- 1 medium-sized cucumber, thinly sliced
- 1/4 cup of bacon bits
- 5 cups of mixed greens, such as romaine lettuce, arugula, swiss chard, mizuna, radicchio
- 1/4 of a red onion, sliced
- For the salad dressing:
- 1/4 cup of apple cider vinegar
- 1/4 cup of virgin olive oil
- 1 teaspoon of salt
- 1/4 cup of honey
- 1/4 cup of Dijon mustard

sssssssssssssssssss

Methods:

Step 1: Prepare the Dressing

In a covered jar, combine apple cider vinegar, virgin olive oil, salt, honey, and Dijon mustard. Close the jar tightly and shake vigorously until all the ingredients are well combined. This homemade dressing brings a delightful balance of sweet, tangy, and savory flavors to the salad.

Step 2: Assemble the Salad

In a large salad bowl, combine the mixed greens, including romaine lettuce, arugula, swiss chard, mizuna, and radicchio. These diverse greens offer a variety of tastes and textures, creating a visually appealing and flavorful salad base.

Step 3: Add Toppings

Thinly slice the cucumber and red onion to add a refreshing crunch and a hint of sharpness to the salad.

Sprinkle shelled sunflower seeds over the greens for a nutty and slightly buttery taste.

Enhance the salad with bacon bits, which contribute a smoky and savory element to the dish.

Step 4: Toss and Serve

Before serving, give the dressing a final shake to ensure all the flavors are well distributed.

Drizzle the desired amount of dressing over the salad and gently toss to coat the greens, toppings, and vegetables evenly.

Fun Facts:

Green salads are a versatile and nutritious dish that can be customized with various ingredients to create a balanced and flavorful meal.

Different types of salad greens offer a variety of textures, flavors, and nutrients.

Suggestions:

Add grilled chicken, shrimp, or tofu to turn this green salad into a complete and satisfying meal.

Experiment with different types of nuts or seeds, such as toasted almonds or pumpkin seeds, for added crunch and nutrition.

30. Celery and Apple Soup

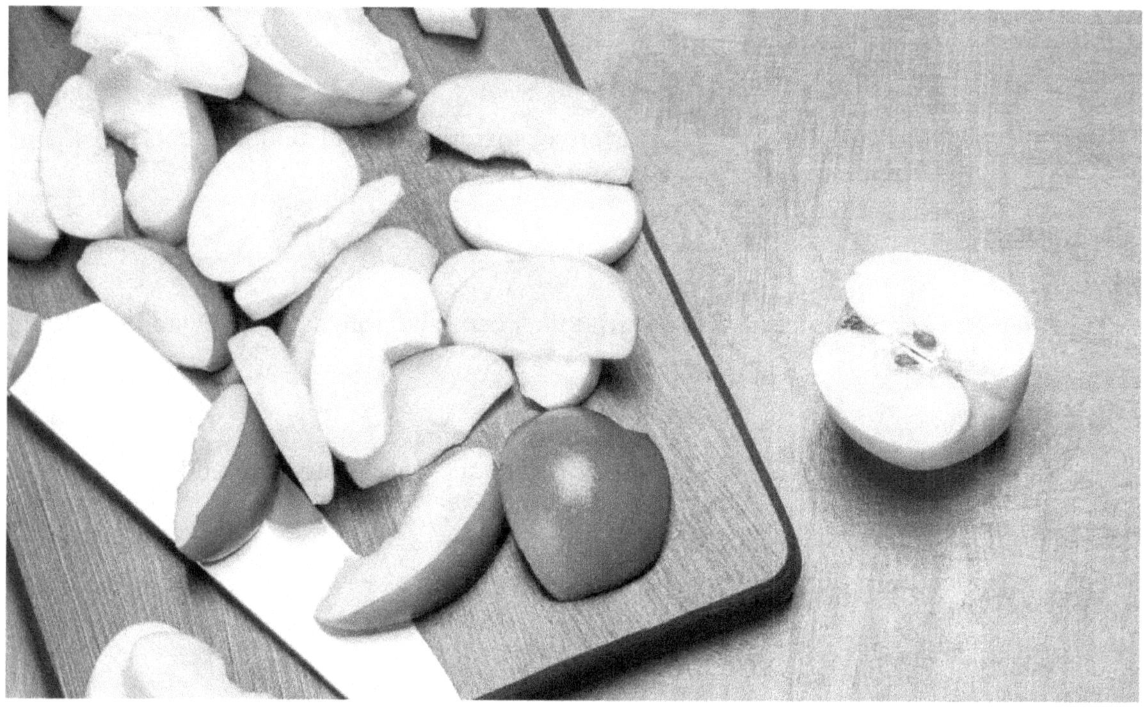

This interesting combination of flavors produces a tasty soup. Remember to serve it with some nice country bread - it would be perfect. The best is to use cooking apples but you can use the other variety too. Keep some bits of apple and celery to garnish the soup in the end.

Serve: 4

Prep Time: 55 minutes

List of Ingredients:

- 1 bay leaf
- 3 sticks of celery, finely chopped
- Salt and pepper
- 2 tablespoons of olive oil
- 1 large onion, finely chopped
- 3 cooking apple, sliced
- 2 pints of vegetable stock

sssssssssssssssssss

Methods:

Step 1: Prepare the Ingredients

Measure out the olive oil, onion, apple, vegetable stock, bay leaf, celery, and seasoning. Having everything ready will streamline the cooking process.

Step 2: Sauté Onion

Warm up the olive oil in a large pan over medium heat. Add the onion and sauté until they become soft and translucent. The gentle cooking ensures a flavorful base for the soup.

Step 3: Add Apple

Introduce the apple to the sautéed onion. Cook for about 3 minutes until the apple begins to soften. The combination of celery and apple offers a delightful balance of flavors.

Step 4: Infuse Flavors

Pour in the vegetable stock and add the bay leaf. This step infuses the soup with depth and complexity while creating a fragrant base for the celery and apple.

Step 5: Incorporate Celery

Add the celery to the pan and season the soup. As the celery cooks, its natural flavors will meld with the other ingredients, enhancing the overall taste.

Step 6: Simmer and Blend

Cover the pan and allow the soup to simmer on medium heat for 30 minutes. This slow simmering allows the ingredients to develop their flavors.

Once done, carefully blend the soup until it reaches a smooth and creamy consistency. An immersion blender or countertop blender can be used for this step.

Step 7: Final Touches

Return the blended soup to the heat and bring it back to a gentle boil. This step ensures that the soup is heated through and ready to be served.

Step 8: Serve and Enjoy

Ladle the hot celery and apple soup into serving bowls. The comforting combination of flavors will make for a delightful and nourishing meal.

Fun Facts:

Celery is a low-calorie vegetable rich in vitamins and minerals, making it a healthy addition to soups.

Apples add a natural sweetness to soups while also providing dietary fiber and antioxidants.

Suggestions:

Garnish the soup with a drizzle of olive oil, a sprinkle of chopped fresh herbs, or a dollop of sour cream for added flavor and visual appeal.

Serve the soup with a side of crusty bread or croutons for a satisfying meal.

31. Asparagus and Greens Salad with Tahini and Poppy Seed Dressing

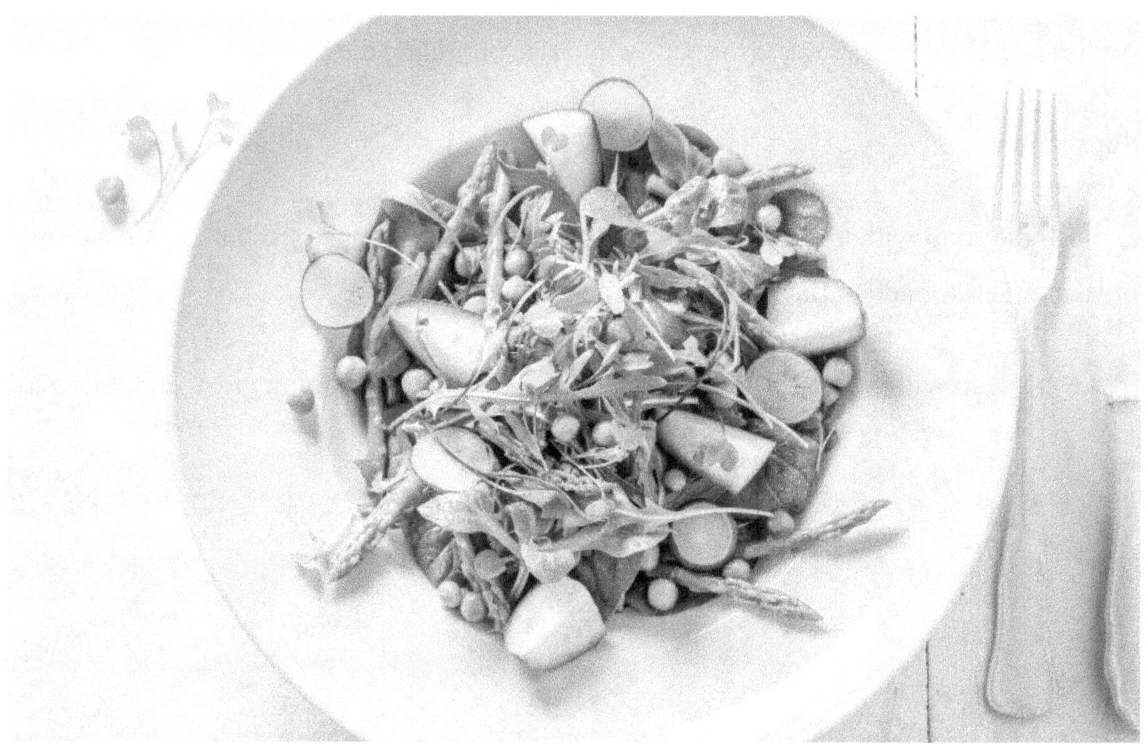

Asparagus can be eaten raw but the texture is not very appealing. It is better to cook it before you eat it. This recipe uses asparagus in a salad along with a very healthy dressing that is made with tahini and poppy seeds.

Serve: 4

Prep Time: 1 hour 10 minutes

List of Ingredients:

For the salad:

- 2 to 3 rainbow carrots, peeled and sliced thinly
- 1 small handful of microgreens, washed well
- 1 small handful of sunflower greens, washed well
- 10 to 12 asparagus stalks, washed well and sliced into ribbons
- 5 radishes, washed well and sliced thinly
- 1 handful of wild spinach

Optional: few pieces of chive blossoms

For the dressing:

- 1 tablespoon of extra-virgin olive oil
- Salt and pepper, to taste
- 2 tablespoons of tahini
- 1 tablespoon of poppy seeds

ssssssssssssssssssss

Methods:

Step 1: Prepare the Dressing

Whisk the extra-virgin olive oil, salt, pepper, tahini, and poppy seeds together in a small bowl. This creates a creamy and flavorful dressing with a delightful crunch from the poppy seeds.

Step 2: Toss the Salad

In a separate bowl, combine the thinly sliced rainbow carrots, microgreens, sunflower greens, sliced asparagus ribbons, thinly sliced radishes, wild spinach, and optional chive blossoms. This variety of greens and vegetables provides a mix of flavors and textures.

Step 3: Drizzle with Dressing

Drizzle the prepared tahini and poppy seed dressing over the salad just before serving. The dressing adds a creamy and nutty element that complements the freshness of the greens and vegetables.

Fun Facts:

Asparagus is a nutrient-rich vegetable known for its distinct flavor and tender texture. It's a great source of vitamins and minerals, including folate and vitamins A, C, and K.

Tahini is a creamy paste made from ground sesame seeds, commonly used in Mediterranean and Middle Eastern cuisines.

Poppy seeds add a delightful crunch and a hint of nutty flavor to dishes, including dressings and baked goods.

Suggestions:

Add grilled chicken, shrimp, or tofu to make this salad a complete and satisfying meal.

Sprinkle some toasted pine nuts or chopped almonds for extra crunch and flavor.

Experiment with different microgreens and baby greens to create a variety of textures and colors in your salad.

32. Spinach Quiche

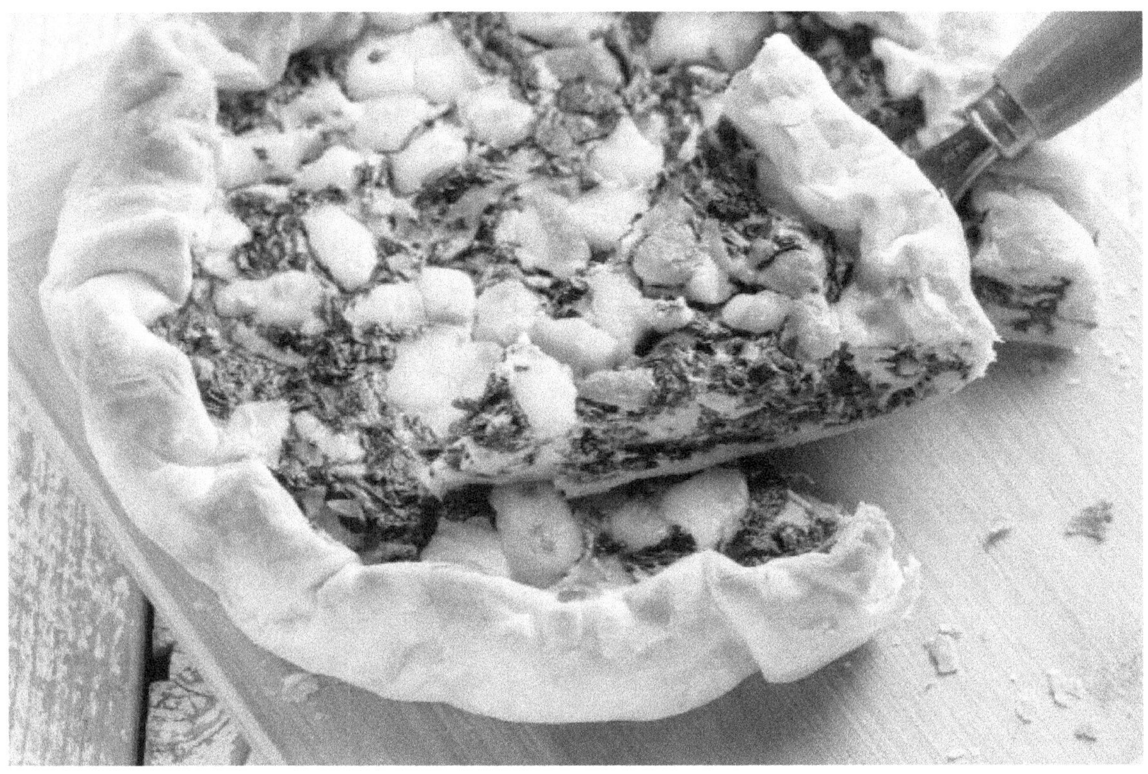

Quiche is a very popular pie. This recipe is full of vegetables that are mixed with eggs and other List of Ingredients. The spinach can make it very sweet or it can be left out for a more savory taste.

Serve: 4

Prep Time: 1 hour 10 minutes

List of Ingredients:

- 1/2 an onion, diced
- 6 cups of spinach, roughly chopped
- 12 eggs
- 1 teaspoon of salt
- 1 teaspoon of pepper
- 1 lb. of breakfast sausage
- 2 cups of mushrooms, sliced
- 1/4 to 1/2 cup of full-fat coconut milk
- 1 teaspoon of garlic powder
- 1 teaspoon of Italian seasoning

sssssssssssssssssss

Methods:

Step 1: Prepare the Ingredients

Begin by dicing half an onion and roughly chopping 6 cups of spinach. These ingredients will contribute to the flavor and texture of the quiche.

Step 2: Cook the Sausage and Vegetables

Heat an oven-safe pan over medium heat and cook the breakfast sausage and diced onion. Stir occasionally until the sausage browns, approximately 7-8 minutes.

Add the sliced mushrooms and cook them with the sausage until they become soft, about 2 minutes. Remove the mixture from the heat.

Step 3: Prepare the Egg Mixture

Crack 12 eggs into a large bowl and add 1/4 to 1/2 cup of full-fat coconut milk. Adjust the amount of coconut milk based on your preference for texture and coconut flavor.

Whisk the eggs and coconut milk together until well blended, creating a light egg mixture.

Step 4: Combine Ingredients

Add the chopped spinach and seasonings to the bowl with the egg mixture.

Incorporate the cooked sausage and mushroom mixture, as well as the rest of the listed ingredients. Mix everything until well combined.

Step 5: Bake the Quiche

Preheat the oven to 400°F and line the oven-safe pan with some of the sausage fat or grease it with oil, butter, or ghee to prevent sticking.

Pour the quiche mixture into the prepared pan and bake for 40-45 minutes or until a knife inserted into the center comes out clean.

Fun Facts:

Quiche is a versatile dish that originated in France and is known for its savory custard filling and flaky pastry crust.

This recipe combines the goodness of eggs, spinach, sausage, and mushrooms to create a flavorful and nutritious quiche.

Quiche can be enjoyed for breakfast, brunch, lunch, or dinner and is often served warm or at room temperature.

Suggestions:

Customize the quiche by adding your favorite ingredients such as bell peppers, cheese, or even different types of cooked meats.

Serve the quiche with a side salad or fresh fruit to create a balanced and satisfying meal.

Quiche can be prepared ahead of time and reheated for a quick and convenient meal option during busy days.

33. Tomato and Pepper Ice

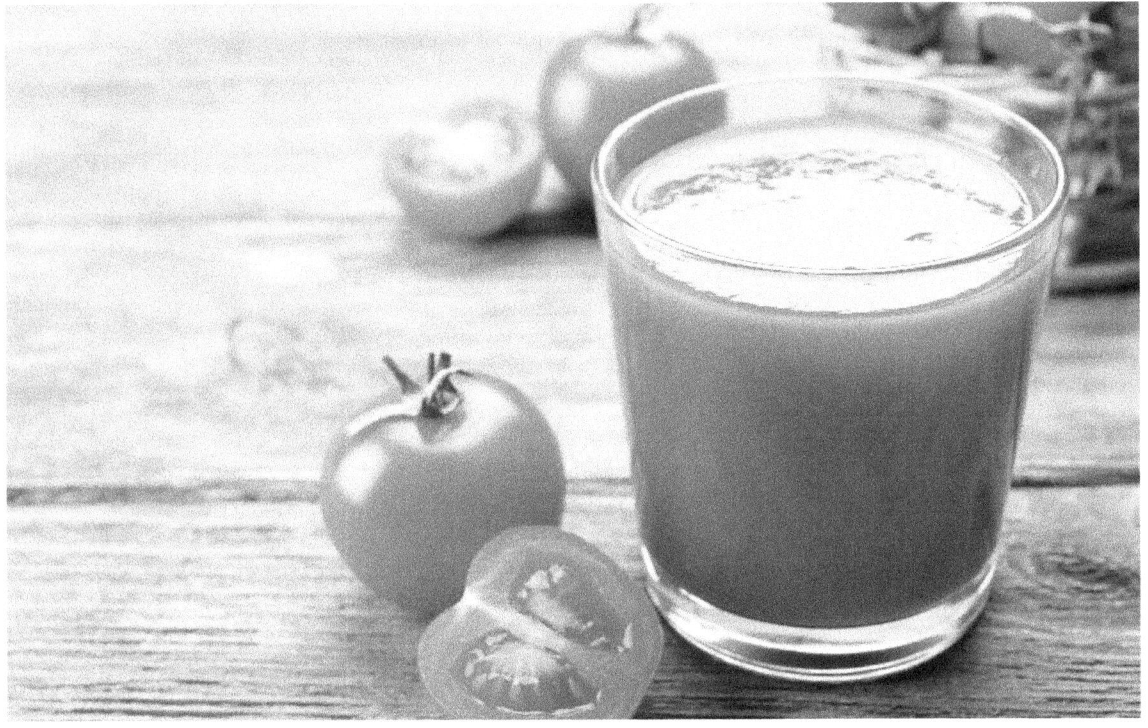

Similar to frozen Gazpacho, this original appetizer is ideal for serving on warm summer days. It could be used in smaller quantities as well, as a palate freshener course to replace conventional sorbet. Be careful not to allow the tomato ice to freeze into a solid block.

Serve: 4

Prep Time: 15 minutes + freezing time

List of Ingredients:

- 6 ice cubes
- 1 red pepper, seeded and finely chopped
- 1 teaspoon of Worcester sauce
- 1 green pepper, seeded and finely chopped
- 4 tomatoes
- Salt and pepper
- ½ cup of tomato juice
- 1 lemon, juiced

sssssssssssssssssss

Methods:

Step 1: Prepare the Tomatoes

Begin by cutting the tops off the tomatoes and setting them aside to use as "hats" later.

Step 2: Scoop and Blend

Gently scoop out the inside of the tomatoes, keeping the pulp and seeds aside.

Place the tomato pulp and seeds in a blender.

Step 3: Blend the Mixture

To the blender, add tomato juice, lemon juice, and Worcestershire sauce.

Break the ice cubes into smaller pieces and add them to the blender as well.

Blend the mixture until it becomes a smooth slush.

Step 4: Freeze and Mash

Pour the slushy mixture into an ice tray and freeze it for about 30 minutes, until it begins to solidify around the edges.

Remove the partially frozen mixture from the tray and mash it to break up the ice crystals.

Step 5: Add Peppers

Mix in the finely chopped green and red peppers with the partially frozen mixture.

Return the mixture to the ice tray and continue freezing for another 1.5 hours, stirring occasionally to prevent it from freezing completely solid.

Step 6: Serve and Enjoy

When ready to serve, allow the mixture to defrost for about 5 minutes. Mash it with a fork to create a slushy texture.

Fill the chilled tomato shells with the slushy mixture and serve immediately.

Fun Facts:

Tomato and Pepper Ice is a unique and refreshing dish that combines the flavors of tomatoes, peppers, and ice, creating a delightful and unexpected treat.

This recipe offers a playful twist on traditional ice-based desserts, incorporating the vibrant colors and flavors of tomatoes and peppers.

Suggestions:

Customize the recipe by using different types of peppers for varying levels of heat and flavor. Consider using bell peppers for a milder taste or spicier peppers like jalapenos for a kick.

Experiment with different herbs and seasonings to enhance the flavor profile. Fresh basil, mint, or a touch of cayenne pepper can add exciting dimensions to the dish.

Garnish the Tomato and Pepper Ice with fresh herbs or a drizzle of balsamic glaze to add a visually appealing and flavorful touch.

Experiment with different types of tomato varieties, such as cherry tomatoes or heirloom tomatoes, for unique visual and taste experiences.

Incorporate a touch of sweetness with a drizzle of pomegranate molasses or raspberry balsamic vinegar.

Fold in a handful of toasted pine nuts or chopped almonds for a nutty crunch.

Create a refreshing contrast by mixing in diced watermelon or cucumber.

Add a touch of umami by incorporating a teaspoon of soy sauce or tamari into the mixture.

For a creamy twist, fold in a tablespoon of plain Greek yogurt or dairy-free yogurt.

Enhance the smokiness by adding a drop or two of liquid smoke to the blended mixture.

Create a tropical fusion by mixing in diced mango or pineapple along with the peppers.

Experiment with different colored bell peppers to create a visually vibrant presentation.

Mix in a pinch of ground coriander or cumin for an exotic and aromatic flavor.

For a burst of sweetness, fold in pomegranate arils or diced strawberries.

Thanks You All!

I am incredibly grateful to you for choosing my book. Each purchase serves as a reminder that people are interested in learning from my experience and expertise, and that fills me with joy.

Out of all the books available on the market, you selected mine, and that is truly special to me. I'm confident that you will find the content of this book helpful and informative, and that it will enhance your culinary skills.

After reading the book, please take a moment to leave your feedback. Even the smallest feedback can help me improve and create better books for my readers. I value the opinions and suggestions of my readers, and I always try to incorporate them in my next works.

Once again, thank you for choosing my book. I hope you enjoy reading it as much as I enjoyed writing it, and that it inspires you to create delicious meals in your kitchen!

Expressing my sincere gratitude,
Ana Rose